SYSTEMIC HEMODYNAMICS AND HEMODYNAMIC MANAGEMENT

B. Bo Sramek, Ph.D.

Copyright © 2002
B. Bo Sramek

All rights reserved. No part of this book may be reproduced in any form, except for the inclusion of brief quotation in review, without permission in writing from the author.

ISBN 1-59196-046-0

Printed in US by Instantpublisher.com

Preface

A healthy body is designed as a perfectly tuned machine. Its cardiovascular system has one overwhelming purpose – to provide an adequate supply of oxygen and nutrients to all tissues. The dynamic modulator of oxygen transport is hemodynamics.

During the second half of the last century, the use of terms "hemodynamics" and "hemodynamic measurement" proliferated. However, these terms started to carry a different meaning within various branches of medicine.

To a general practitioner, hemodynamic measurement represented measurement of a patient's arterial blood pressure, maybe the heart rate.

A cardiologist was driven by a hemodynamic need to measure blood pressures in vasculature and heart chambers, and to obtain information about the heart performance, such as assessing myocardial contractility and measuring ejection fraction.

To an anesthesiologist or intensivist, hemodynamic measurement represented an expressed task to catheterize a patient with a flow-directed, pulmonary artery catheter to obtain values of filling pressures of the left and right heart and Cardiac Output (CO).

To a medical equipment manufacturer, attaching the word "hemodynamic" become a code name indicating a cardiovascular significance of their device. Any instrument involved in monitoring heart rate or blood pressure became a "hemodynamic monitor."

While over the last fifty years these "hemodynamic" patient monitors have undergone tremendous technological improvements, the **outcomes** of patients monitored by these devices have not changed considerably over the same time period. The reasons are simple: These monitors, actually, have not monitored hemodynamics, as we understand it today. The monitoring "hemodynamic" modalities were not selected as a result of expressed intellectual need to manage patients into a desired hemodynamic state and, therefore, improve their outcomes. These modalities were incorporated into patient monitors as a result of their historical availability: Displaying the ECG signal and resulting digital value of Heart Rate (HR) were the first parameters to be implemented. Then, when oscillometric technique matured, the Systolic/Diastolic (S/D) and Mean Arterial Pressure (MAP) were added to the monitoring armament. After the pulse oximetry and respiration bioimpedance techniques were perfected, the Percentage Saturation of Oxygen in Arterial Blood (SpO_2) and Respiratory Rate (RR) completed the list of displayed digital parameters by noninvasive patient monitors. Obviously, invasive measurements of blood pressures in vessels and heart chambers and invasive measurement of CO were subsequently added to monitors' capabilities, however, these features have not been routinely used on every patient. Since only adequate values of CO and related adequate levels of Oxygen Delivery (DO_2) correlate with survival, the explanation of poor outcomes becomes clear.

A link between current patient monitors and poor outcomes of patients monitored by these devices is the monitors' philosophy: "The purpose of the monitor is to obtain an early warning of an impending (cardiovascular) disaster." Monitors have, therefore, alarms, which the clinician sets as to obtain an alarm signal when the monitored parameter exceeds the preset range. However, the monitored parameter has to enter the "gray zone" in which the patient is probably already compromised and the clinician is forced into "putting out fires" rather than maintaining the patient in a desired hemodynamic state, which would be conducive to rapid healing, fast recovery and shorter hospital stay.

In addition to semantic and conceptual problems described above, there are much deeper intellectual problems with current hemodynamics:

- Understanding hemodynamics is incomplete and, in some of its parts, incorrect.
- There is no expressed need to determine adequacy of perfusion in every patient.
- Most of clinical decisions are based upon blood pressure measurement only.
- There has been a continuous quest to identify just a single parameter that is supposed to describe the status of the entire cardiovascular system (such as the perceived importance of ejection fraction measurement).
- Drugs for treatment of hemodynamic disorders are designed and described as vehicles for treatment of a single parameter (such as the antihypertensive drugs).

These misconceptions have created a culture that tends to treat a hemodynamic **symptom,** rather than seeking to identify the **causes** of abnormal hemodynamics and finding the therapy for a patient, which will result in normovolemia, normoinotropy and normovasoactivity, because only such a patient can be normotensive and normodynamic. When normochronotropy is then therapeutically established as well, he will also have an adequate perfusion blood flow. And only a patient with adequate supply of oxygen to all tissues can be called healthy in respect to the primary function of cardiovascular system - transport of oxygen.

This textbook will:
- Re-define hemodynamics as blood pressure-blood flow relationships, acquired simultaneously.
- Debunk the myths of current "per-minute," or "steady-state" systemic hemodynamics and introduce the reader to the physiologically correct concepts of "per-beat" hemodynamics.
- Define the physiologic and mathematic relationships between the hemodynamic modulators (intravascular volume, inotropy and vasoactivity) and their modulat-

ing consequence – the systemic hemodynamic state (i.e., mean blood pressure and blood flow values over one heart beat interval).
- Separate the hemodynamic modulation from the perfusion flow modulation, performed via chronotropic compensation by HR.
- Explain why, when and how the cardiac output should be measured to underscore the importance of this perfusion blood flow parameter as the only **dynamic** modulator of oxygen delivery.
- Define the therapeutic goal as the desired hemodynamic, perfusion blood flow and oxygen delivery states.
- Present four different therapeutic goals for four different subgroups of patients:
    (a) Neonates and pediatrics,
    (b) Adult males and postmenopausal females,
    (c) Gravidas and nongravidas, and
    (d) Surgical patients in the immediate postoperative period.
- Redirect the current focus on cardiovascular system from "arterial blood pressure and/or ECG signal generator" to its real function – a vehicle for oxygen transport.
- Change the definition of cardiovascular health from current focus on normotension, to adequate delivery of oxygen to all tissues under all metabolic states, while, at the same time, maintaining normotension.
- Demonstrate how to manage each patient into a normohemodynamic and normoperfusion state (therapeutic goal), thus changing the concept of cardiovascular medicine from **reactive** (the patient is treated when his hemodynamic disorder is diagnosed and/or demonstrates itself) to **proactive** (maintaining the patient within his specific therapeutic goal).

B. Bo Sramek, Chairman
International Hemodynamic Society
(www.hemodynamicsociety.org)

Contents

Preface	3
1. Introduction.	10
2. Cardiac Output – Oxygen Transport Dynamic Modulator: Why, When and How it should be Measured	13
3. Oxygen Transport: O_2 Delivery and O_2 Consumption . .	30
4. Hemodynamic Modulation: Per minute or per beat? . .	33
4.1. Concepts of Per-minute Hemodynamics	33
4.2. Concepts of Per-beat Hemodynamics .	45
4.2.1 Hemodynamic Modulators . .	53
4.2.1.1 Preload: Intravascular Volume Modulation	53
4.2.1.2 Myocardial Contractility: Mechanical & Pharmacological Modulation . . .	54
4.2.1.3 Afterload: Vasoactivity Modulation	61
4.2.2 Perfusion Blood Flow: Chronotropy Modulation . .	62
4.2.3 Timing Considerations of Hemodynamic Modulation . . .	64

5. Hemodynamic Management . . 65

    5.1. Graphical Presentation of Hemodynamic State: The Hemodynamic Map . 65

    5.2. Hemodynamic Effects of Vasoactivity . 67

    5.3. Hemodynamic Effects of Intravascular Volume and Inotropy . 71

    5.4. The Hemodynamic Management Chart 75

    5.5. Hemodynamic Responses to Hemodynamic and Perfusion Blood Flow Management 78

        5.5.1. Calculations of Percentage Deviations in Volume, Inotropy, Vasoactivity and Chronotropy from their Respective Ideal Values 80

            5.5.1.1. Calculation of Percentage Deviation in Inotropy . . 80

            5.5.1.2. Calculation of Percentage Deviation in Intravascular Volume . . 81

            5.5.1.3. Calculation of Percentage Deviation in Vasoactivity . . . 82

            5.5.1.4. Calculation of Percentage Deviation in Chronotropy . . . 83

6. Normal Hemodynamic, O_2 Delivery and TEB Values in Neonatal and Pediatric Patients . 85

7. Normal Hemodynamic, O_2 Delivery and TEB
   Values in Gravidas and Nongravidas . 94

8. Hemodynamic Management with "Per-beat"
   Hemodynamics: Case Studies . . 100

   8.1. Hemodynamic Management of a Surgical
        Patient in the ICU 100

   8.2. Hemodynamic Management of a
        Hypertensive Patient . . . 109

References 119

Index 122

1. Introduction

"Hemodynamics is concerned with the forces generated by the heart and the resulting motion of blood through the cardiovascular system" (W.R. Milnor: Hemodynamics, Williams & Wilkins, 1982).

The above-stated definition clearly identifies the purpose of the cardiovascular system as the blood motion, i.e., oxygen and nutrients delivery system, and hemodynamics as a physical and physiological base to accomplish this task. Since the forces generated by the heart demonstrate themselves to an outside observer (clinician) as the blood flow/blood pressure relationships, hemodynamics deals with these inseparable flow/pressure pairs at different nodes of the cardiovascular system. Blood flow is the hemodynamic cause; blood pressure is the hemodynamic consequence, formed across the resistance and compliance of vasculature or, in chambers, as a result of chamber compliance. Utilizing blood pressure measurements for clinical decisions, such as, for instance, use of PAOP (Pulmonary Artery Occluded Pressure) to assess volemia/preload, carries a significant risk of misinformation and resulting misdiagnoses: When measuring PAOP, the only parameter accurately measured is the PAOP. However, inferring the level of intravascular volume from the value of PAOP may be profoundly misleading[7]: Blood volume and PAOP are related to each other through an unknown compliance of heart chambers. A young patient with compliant chambers can be volume overloaded while having a "normal" PAOP; in contrast, an older patient with a stiff ventricle can be profoundly hypovolemic, while the measured PAOP is within a "normal" range.

We will be concentrating in this textbook on **systemic hemodynamics** – blood flow/blood pressure relationship at the output node of the left heart. The focus on systemic hemodynamics is justified - dysfunction or malfunction of systemic hemodynamics is the major contributor to a lower quality of life and a shorter life span of many in- and outpatients anywhere in the world.

The heart is a pulsatile pump, delivering blood into the aorta in boluses during each ejection period; it is disconnected from the vasculature during the diastolic phase due to a closed aortic valve. The aortic pressure is, therefore, pulsatile as well (see Fig.1.1). Its highest (systolic) level corresponds to the largest integrated volume of blood delivered to the aorta during each ejection phase. Due to compliance of arterial system, arterial blood pressure signal does not copy the blood flow. Blood stored in distended and slowly shrinking arteries during each diastole, causes the pressure to decay only to the diastolic level, till the next ejection phase repeats the process. The systolic blood pressure level is a function of volume and viscosity of blood ejected, rate of contraction of myocardium (myocardial contractility) and arterial impedance. On the other hand, the diastolic level is a function of volume and viscosity of blood ejected, and the vascular resistance.

Though study of instantaneous values of aortic blood pressure and blood flow is of interest to a cardiovascular physiologist (to derive the value of vascular impedance as a function of time), we will concentrate in our pursuit of systemic hemodynamics on **mean values of blood flow and blood pressure over one heartbeat interval**, since only these carry the **clinical significance.** Fig.1.1 describes the interrelationship of blood flow through the aortic valve and the aortic blood pressure over one heart beat interval. The hemodynamically significant blood flow, therefore, is the **Stroke Volume (SV)** – a mean value of blood flow over one heartbeat interval. SV represents a steady-state blood flow level, which the left ventricle would deliver into the aorta if the heart would be a constant flow delivery device and not a pulsatile pump. The hemodynamically significant blood pressure is the **Mean Arterial Pressure (MAP)** – a mean value of aortic blood pressure over one heartbeat interval. MAP is an aortic blood pressure, which would exist in the aorta if the heart would be a constant flow delivery device and not a pulsatile pump.

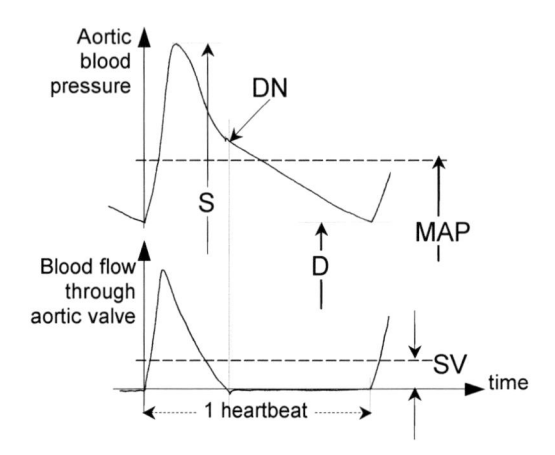

Fig.1.1 A relationship between aortic blood pressure and blood flow through aortic valve. Systolic (S), Diastolic (D) pressure levels indicated. Mean Arterial Pressure (MAP) is the mean level of aortic blood pressure over one heartbeat interval. DN indicates dicrotic notch – the end of ejection phase. SV indicates Stroke Volume – a mean value of blood flow over one heartbeat interval. MAP and SV would exist in cardiovascular system if heart would be a constant flow delivery device and not a pulsatile pump.

While understanding hemodynamics as blood flow/blood pressure relationships, we may not loose our focus on the primary purpose of hemodynamics - it is its blood flow component, which is the dynamically responding vehicle for delivery of oxygen as to satisfy continually changing dynamics of oxygen demand of all tissues. The next chapter will deal with this aspect.

2. Cardiac Output – O_2 Transport Dynamic Modulator: Why, When and How it should be Measured

There seems to be a split opinion within the medical community about the importance of Cardiac Output (CO) - the global blood flow:

On one hand, Braunwald[1] calls CO "the ultimate expression of cardiovascular performance." According to him, CO is one of the most important hemodynamic/perfusion base assessment parameters, related to a true definition of cardiovascular health. On the other hand, many physicians have left medical schools with a belief that normal value of Cardiac Output in an adult human is CO_{normal} = 5.5 l/min, its determination is unimportant in outpatients and in a majority of inpatients, and its measurement is of value only in high risk and/or critically ill patients.

What are the facts?

The primary function of the cardiovascular system is transport of oxygen. In O_2 transport, blood is the vehicle oxygen is the cargo. This should lead us to the conclusion that an adequate O_2 delivery to all organs under all metabolic conditions is the only true definition of cardiovascular health.

Global O_2 Delivery (DO_2) [ml/min] is a blood flow and not blood pressure-related parameter:

$$DO_2 = CO \times 10\, Hgb \times SaO_2 \times 1.34 \qquad [Eq.2.1]$$

where:
Hgb is hemoglobin [g/dl];
  (normal range of Hgb: men 14<Hgb<18 [g/dl], women 12<Hgb<16 [g/dl])[3]
SaO_2 is percentage saturation of O_2 in arterial blood [%]
1.34 is the O_2 affinity to hemoglobin constant
  (1g of hemoglobin binds 1.34 ml of O_2)

In a patient who is not hemorrhaging (Hgb is constant) and with normally functioning lungs (SaO$_2$ is close to 100%, i.e., another constant) CO thus is the only dynamic modulator in the O$_2$ delivery equation (Eq.2.1) above. Under these conditions, normal value of CO then equates to normal DO$_2$.

Milnor[2] documents that normal CO in all resting, supine, normo-weight mammals is a linear function of their weight at approx. 0.1 l/min/kg (see Fig.2.1).

Normal CO = 5.5 l/min for all resting adults is, therefore, a fallacy, since CO = 5.5 l/min can be a normal value for normoweight, 55 kg woman only. In order to determine if CO of a given patient is within its normal range, CO must be indexed by a parameter related to the patient's body mass. Only indexed blood flow parameters exhibit one normal range.

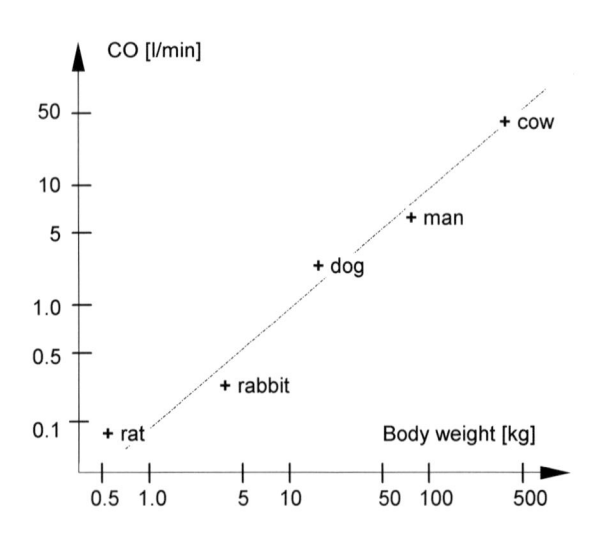

Fig.2.1. Relation between CO and body weight in different mammalian species. From Milnor WR: Hemodynamics. Williams & Wilkins, 1982, p 155

Indexing CO by Body Surface Area (BSA), though not perfect[2], has become a clinical standard, since it takes in an account the variation of subject's weight from ideal. **Cardiac Index (CI)**, a global blood flow per minute, is defined as:

$$\mathbf{CI = CO/BSA} \qquad [Eq.2.2]$$

where:
CI is Cardiac Index [l/min/m^2]
and

$$\mathbf{BSA = W^{0.425} \times H^{0.725} \times 0.007184} \qquad [Eq.2.2a]$$

(DuBois & DuBois Formula[14])
where W is weight [kg] and H is height [cm]

Normal CI for resting, supine adults[3] is

$$\mathbf{CI_{normal} = 3.5 \ l/min/m^2 \pm 20\%} \qquad [Eq.2.3]$$

While indexing global blood flow, Global O₂ Delivery has to be indexed as well. The **Global O₂ Delivery Index (DO₂I)** is, therefore, defined as:

$$\mathbf{DO_2I = CI \times 10 \ Hgb \times SaO_2 \times 1.34} \qquad [Eq.2.4]$$

Normal Global DO₂I for resting, supine adults is

$$\mathbf{DO_2I_{normal} = 660 \ ml/min/m^2 \pm 25\%} \qquad [Eq.2.5]$$

(an increased range from 20% in CI to 25% in DO₂I is due to difference of Hgb between men and women – see Eq.2.1 for Hgb values).

It is a common knowledge from cardiovascular physiology that

$$\mathbf{CI = (SI \times HR)/1000} \qquad [Eq.2.6]$$

where:
SI is Stroke Index [ml/beat/m^2] and
HR is Heart Rate [beats/min]
1000 is a constant to convert ml (milliliters) into l (liters)

Similarly to CI, SI (the global blood flow per beat) has to be indexed to obtain a normal range. Normal **Stroke Index (SI)** for supine, resting adults is[3]:

$$SI_{normal} = SV/BSA = 47 \text{ ml/beat/m}^2 \pm 34\% \quad [Eq.2.7]$$

In a healthy, young adult, CI increases 500% between rest and strenuous physical exercise. The chronotropic modulation by HR typically provides for a 300% contribution (from HR = 60 beats/min at rest to HR = 180 beats/min at peak exercise), while the remaining 66% is the result of augmentation of SI by hemodynamic modulating effects of intravascular volume, inotropy and vasoactivity[4]. See the augmentation process as a function of HR in Fig.2.2 below:

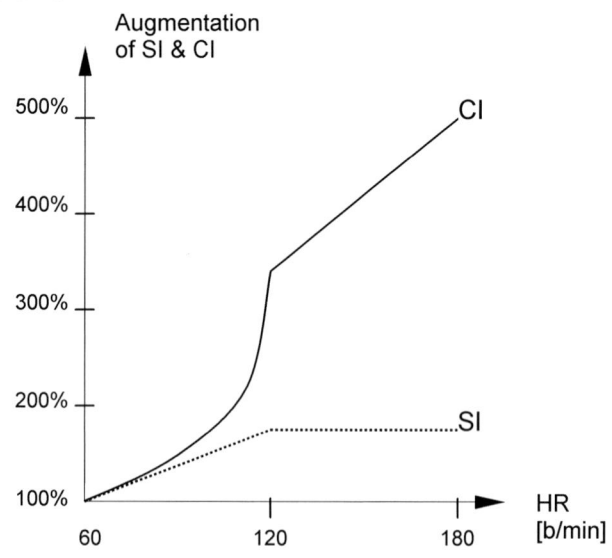

Fig.2.2. Augmentation of SI and CI in response to an increased oxygen demand as a function of HR

At a peak exercise, normal values of CI and SI, therefore, are:

$$CI_{normal} = 17.5 \text{ l/min/m}^2 \pm 20\% \quad [Eq.2.8]$$

and

$$SI_{normal} = 78 \text{ ml/beat/m}^2 \pm 34\% \quad [Eq.2.9]$$

The heart is, therefore, both a variable frequency and variable volumetric output device; it augments its volumetric output till the HR ≅ 120 b/min, at which frequency it becomes a constant output volume device; additional perfusion needs are fulfilled only by a chronotropic compensation by HR.

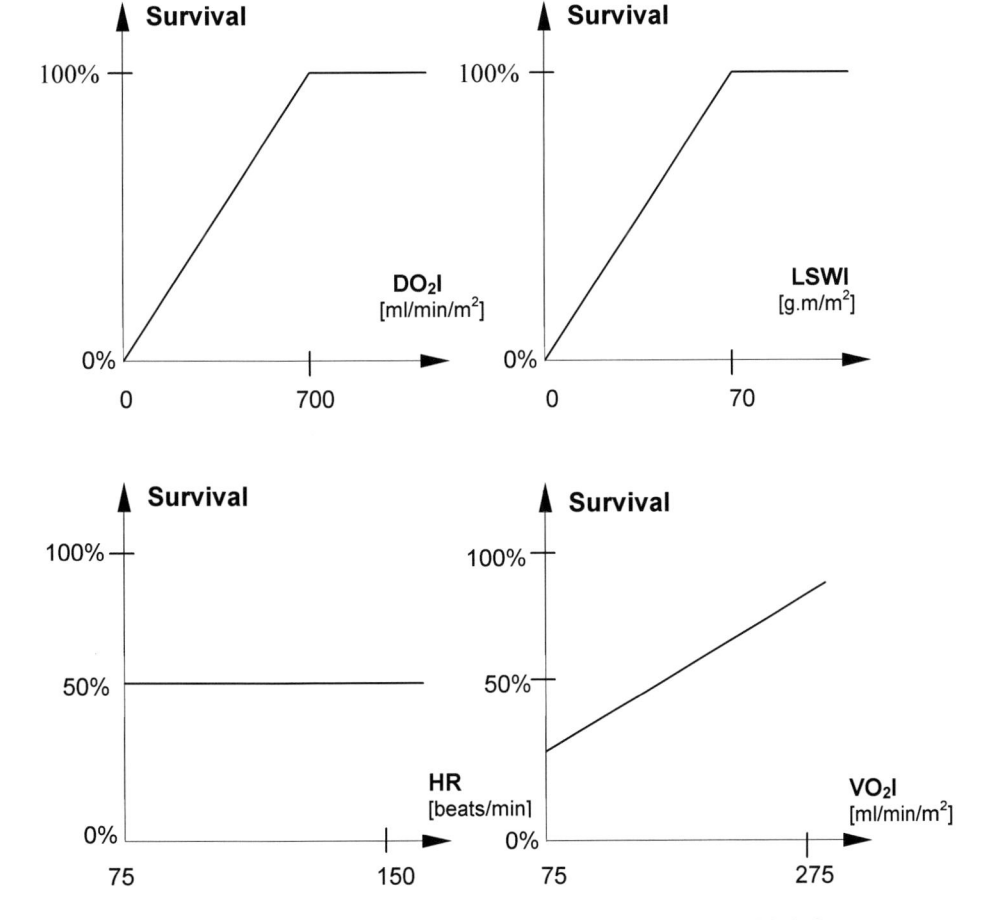

Fig.2.3: Survival of surgical patients after a major surgery as a function of their Oxygen Delivery Index (DO$_2$I), Left Stroke Work Index (LSWI), Heart Rate (HR) and Oxygen Consumption Index (VO$_2$I) in the immediate postoperative period (1-36 hour postoperatively). From Shoemaker WC, et al. Therapy of critically ill postoperative patients based on outcome prediction and prospective clinical trials; The Surgical Clinics of North America, August 1985, Critical Care, WB Saunders Co., p 811

In the '80s, a group or California researchers[5] studied retrospectively the relationships between the survival of patients after a major surgery and values of hemodynamic parameters, obtained from an extensive invasive monitoring using catheters during the postoperative period. The graphs in Fig.2.3 on preceding page, published in this study, show that only two parameters (DO_2I and LSWI) correlated strongly with survival. Survival of these patients, though, steadily increasing with an increase in Global Oxygen Consumption Index (VO_2I), was totally unrelated to postoperative heart rate (HR). They also documented the time dependency of survival-related parameters: DO_2I and LSWI had to be maintained **above the survival threshold levels** during the **first 36 postoperative hours** to assure 100% survivals.

In summary, the conditions for postoperative survival can be expressed as:

$$DO_2I \geq 700 \text{ ml/min/m}^2 \quad\quad [Eq.2.10]$$

and

$$LSWI \geq 70 \text{ g.m/m}^2 \quad\quad [Eq.2.11]$$

where:
LSWI is the Left Stroke Work Index [g.m/m^2]

The Left Stroke Work Index is defined as[4]:

$$LSWI = 0.0144 \text{ (MAP} - \text{LAP)/SI} \quad\quad [Eq.2.12]$$

where:
MAP is the Mean Arterial Pressure [Torr]; [1 Torr = 1 mm Hg]
LAP is the Left Atrial Pressure [Torr]; LAP = (PAOP-2),
where PAOP [Torr] is the Pulmonary Artery Occluded Pressure

This study established a strong correlation between supranormal level of perfusion blood flow and oxygen transport in the immediate postoperative period and survival. Normal level of postoperative CI had to be increased to:

$$CI_{\text{normal postop}} \geq 4.5 \text{ l/min/m}^2 \pm 20\% \qquad [\text{Eq.2.13}]$$

Analyzing Eqs.2.10-13, we can conclude that the relationship between LSWI and survival corresponds to a normotension (MAP = 85 Torr $\pm$ 22%, and LAP = 6 Torr $\pm$ 22%)[3] and a 20% augmentation of SI to a level SI$\geq$56 ml/beat/m².

The reported[5] "supranormal" levels of DO_2I, VO_2I and CI actually represent **normal** perfusion levels for the postoperative state: Under these conditions, all organs are adequately perfused as before the surgery, plus the additional oxygen delivery is directed to the surgical wound.

This statement can be rephrased the following way:

In a surgical patient, who is not hemodynamically and perfusion flow compromised (has the hemodynamic modulators in the postoperative period at their respective normal levels – i.e., normovolemia, normoinotropy, normovasoactivity + normochronotropy), an increased O_2 demand is met by a spontaneous augmentation of SI and an increase in HR as to (a) to maintain perfusion of all organs at their normal, preoperative level, **plus** (b) to fulfill the additional and preferential perfusion needs of the new, temporary organ – the surgical wound. This patient then becomes a survivor.

In contrast, in a patient who is hemodynamically and perfusion flow compromised as a result of surgery (hypovolemia and/or hypoinotropy and/or vasoconstriction and/or hypochronotropy), the preferential perfusion needs of the surgical wound are met at the expense of **reduced** blood flow to other organs. Depending on the level of their perfusion deficiency, and if this state lasts more than 36 hours postoperatively, the organs inadequately perfused will start failing and the patient dies in approximately 92 hours postoperatively from a single or multiple organ failure.

Currently, there are two methods for measurement of CI, which have become clinically accepted: Thermodilution (TD), and Thoracic Electrical Bioimpedance (TEB):

Thermodilution Technique (TD)

The principle of the thermodilution technique is based upon Stewart-Hamilton Law[6]: If an indicator of a known concentration is injected into a flowing fluid (the flow must be **laminar and nonpulsatile** to achieve an even mixture of indicator-fluid), then the variation of concentration of indicator as a function of time taken downstream from the injection point is indicative of the flow rate, which had to be responsible for the indicator dilution.

In TD, a multi-lumen, balloon-tipped catheter is inserted into the jugular or subclavian vein and, when the balloon is partially inflated, floated through the superior vena cava, right atrium and right ventricle all the way so its tip ends in a pulmonary artery. The indicator is a bolus of chilled, or room temperature saline or dextrose injected into the blood stream through a port of the catheter located in a vicinity of right atrium. Detection of the temperature of the indicator-blood mixture is performed by a thermistor located at the tip of the catheter in pulmonary artery. The TD curve and the CO_{TD} equation are in Fig.2.4.

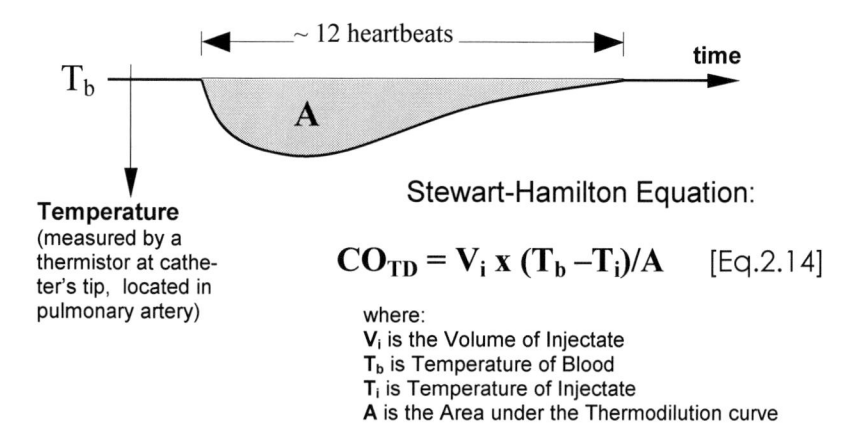

Fig.2.4. Stewart-Hamilton indicator dilution principle: Temperature plot of a blood-injectate mixture measured in pulmonary artery after injecting bolus of a lower temperature injectate into the blood stream in the vicinity of right atrium

Stewart-Hamilton Equation:

$$CO_{TD} = V_i \times (T_b - T_i)/A \quad [Eq.2.14]$$

where:
V_i is the Volume of Injectate
T_b is Temperature of Blood
T_i is Temperature of Injectate
A is the Area under the Thermodilution curve

A computer attached externally to the thermistor leads calculates CO_{TD} according to Eq.2.14. A continuous CO_{TD} using an upstream blood warming as an indicator has been introduced recently.

One feature of a TD catheter has been heralded as its major clinical advantage: A pressure gage attached to one of the lumens of the catheter, which extends all the way to its tip, measures continuously the Pulmonary Artery Pressure (PAP) and, when the balloon is inflated and occludes the pulmonary artery, the Pulmonary Artery Occluded Pressure (PAOP) can be measured. PAOP closely relates to LAP (LAP ≅ PAOP − 2 Torr)[4] and, according to the catheter's manufacturers, thus relates to preload. However, the level of preload (i.e., intravascular volume) is related to LAP through an unknown ventricular compliance and may be misleading[7].

TD requires a sterile environment, a skilled clinician for the catheter insertion and a skilled staff for CO determinations. Its clinical accuracy is 15-20%[6]. TD overestimates low CO in humans[17]. TD technique is fairly expensive[8]. It also is risky: TD mortality rates are up to 4% and morbidity up to 53%[9,10].

Thoracic Electrical Bioimpedance (TEB)

The term bioimpedance (Z) relates to the resistance of body tissues to a high frequency (HF), low magnitude electrical current. The principle of this technique is based upon the fact that blood is the most electrically conductive substance in the body. Fig.2.5 depicts the electrodes' location.

The measurement current passes between two pairs of electrodes located on the upper neck and upper abdomen in a direction parallel with the spine. It seeks the shortest and the most conductive pathway. Since the alveoli in the lungs are filled with non-conductive air, the majority of the TEB measurement current flows through the thoracic aorta and superior and inferior vena cava.

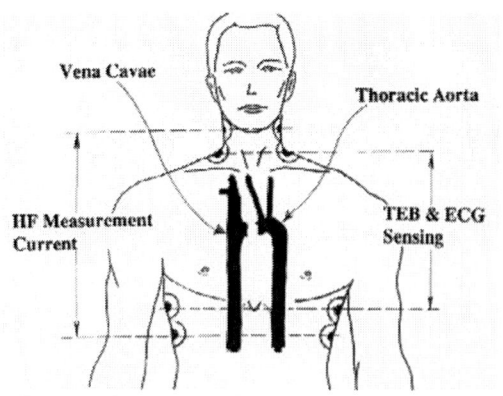

Fig.2.5: Placement of TEB electrodes on landmarks of neck and thorax (HF = high frequency).

Four sensing electrodes are placed along the frontal plane at the levels delineating the thorax (the root of the neck and the diaphragm). These four sensing electrodes detect both the ECG signals and the HF voltage, developed across the thorax, which is proportional to thoracic impedance. The thorax acts as an impedance transducer. The steady-state level of TEB (Z_0 = Base Impedance) is indirectly proportional to thoracic fluids content (TFC = 1/Z₀, where TFC is the Thoracic Fluids Conductivity [Ω^{-1}],). Blood tidal variations due to respiration are the sources of respiratory signal (ΔZ_{resp}), from which respiratory rate is determined.

An important aspect of TEB is the origin of its cardiovascular signal, explained in Fig.2.6 on a section of thoracic aorta:

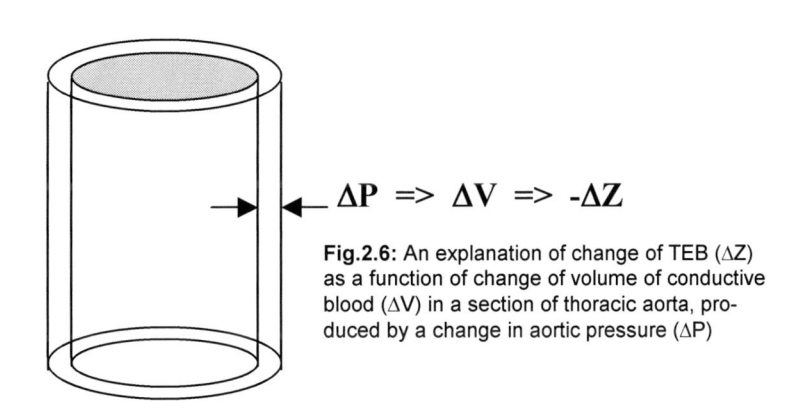

$$\Delta P \Rightarrow \Delta V \Rightarrow -\Delta Z$$

Fig.2.6: An explanation of change of TEB (ΔZ) as a function of change of volume of conductive blood (ΔV) in a section of thoracic aorta, produced by a change in aortic pressure (ΔP)

An increase in arterial pressure ΔP results in displacement of the aortic wall, producing an increase in aortic volume by ΔV, which, in return, results in -ΔZ (aorta, holding more blood, becomes more conductive). ΔZ is measured by TEB. With a compliant aorta, these plethysmographic changes over time are images of arterial blood pressure signal (see dZ = ΔZ in Fig.2.7):

$$\Delta P \Rightarrow \Delta V \Rightarrow -\Delta Z \quad [\text{Eq.2.15}]$$
$$[\text{Torr}] \quad [\text{ml}] \quad [\Omega]$$

An interesting physical aspect of TEB becomes obvious, when, instead of changes of these variables, we examine their rates of their changes over time:

$$dP/dt \Rightarrow dV/dt \Rightarrow dZ/dt \quad [\text{Eq.2.16}]$$
$$[\text{Torr/sec}] \quad [\text{ml/sec}] \quad [\Omega/\text{sec}]$$

The dZ/dt signal, which TEB processes by electronic differentiation of ΔZ, is, actually, an image of aortic volume change in time, i.e., dZ/dt signal is an image of aortic blood flow (see dZ/dt in Fig.2.7). However, there is another, non-plethysmographic component of the TEB signal: Due to a velocity-related alignment of erythrocytes with the main axis of aorta, blood's conductivity is increasing with an increasing velocity of blood as well[11, 18]. The resulting TEB signal thus is a sum of both plethysmographic and velocity components.

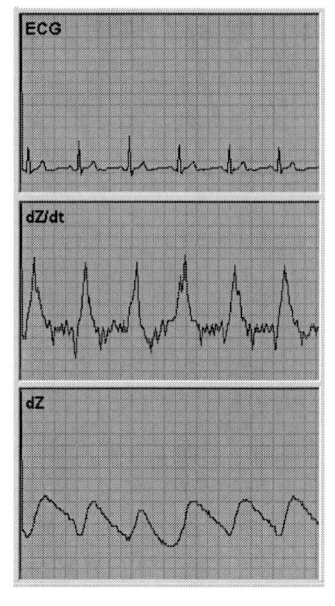

Fig.2.7. TEB-obtained signals of ECG, dZ/dt, ΔZ (marked as dZ) as displayed by HOTMAN® B100 System. (Courtesy HEMO SAPIENS® INC.)

When dZ/dt is normalized by the Base Impedance, Z_o, the resulting TEB-measured parameter, called the **Ejection Phase Contractility Index (EPCI)**, becomes a noninvasive measure of ejection phase contractility. EPCI is defined as

$$\mathbf{EPCI = (dZ/dt)_{max}/Z_o} \quad [sec^{-1}] \qquad [Eq.2.17a]$$

or

$$\mathbf{EPCI = (dZ/dt)_{max} \times TFC} \qquad [Eq.2.17b]$$

(see the discussion on myocardial contractility in Chapter 4.2.1.2).

If dZ/dt is an image of aortic blood flow, then its second derivative, d^2Z/dt^2, represents the acceleration of aortic blood flow. Its peak value, $(d^2Z/dt^2)_{max}$, normalized by Z_o, is a direct, and noninvasive measure if inotropic state, called the **Inotropic State Index (ISI)**.

ISI is defined as

$$\mathbf{ISI = (d^2Z/dt^2)_{max}/Z_o} \qquad [\text{sec}^{-2}] \qquad [\text{Eq.2.18a}]$$

or as

$$\mathbf{ISI = (d^2Z/dt^2)_{max} \times TFC} \qquad [\text{Eq.2.18b}]$$

(see the discussion related to inotropy in Chapter 4.2.1.2)

Since the sensing electrodes also detect the ECG signal, then the Systolic Time Intervals (Pre-ejection Period, PEP [sec], and the Ventricular Ejection Time, VET [sec]) can be measured from the Q-time of the ECG QRS complex and prominent landmarks on dZ/dt signal, which correspond to opening and closure of aortic valve. $(dZ/dt)_{max}$ then represents the Aortic Peak Flow (see Fig.4.2.3).

The Systolic Time Intervals contain important information about the mechanical performance of the ventricle, as related to Ejection Fraction (EF), documented by Capan et al[15]. Ejection Fraction (EF) can be estimated from Capan's Equation[15]. See Fig.4.2.4 for normal STI values.

$$\mathbf{EF \cong 0.84 - 0.64 \, (PEP/VET)} \qquad [\text{Eq.2.19}]$$

where:
PEP is the Pre-Ejection Period [sec]
VET is the Ventricular Ejection Time [sec]

SV [ml/beat] is calculated from Sramek's Equation[11,12,18]:

$$\mathbf{SV = VEPT_{gender} \times VET \times EPCI} \qquad [\text{Eq.2.20}]$$

where:
$VEPT_{gender}$ is the Volume of Electrically Participating Tissue [ml]
    (see following text on next page for an explanation of $VEPT_{gender}$)
VET is the Ventricular Ejection Time [sec]

$EPCI = (dZ/dt)_{max}/Z_o = (dZ/dt)_{max} \times TFC$
where
Z_0 is the Base Impedance [Ω];
Note that modern TEB devices display TFC = $1/Z_0$, since TFC (Thoracic Fluid Conductivity) parallels the content of thoracic fluids

Directly measured parameters by TEB are:
- TFC = $1/Z_o$ [Ω^{-1}]
- $(dZ/dt)_{max}$ [Ω/sec]
- $(d^2Z/dt^2)_{max}$ [Ω/sec^{-2}]
- HR [b/min] derived from R-R intervals of the ECG signal
- VET [sec]
- RR (Respiratory Rate) [breaths/min], derived from respiratory component of TEB signal

The following calculations are performed automatically by the TEB system:
- VEPT [ml] is calculated from Eq.2.23
- EPCI [sec^{-1}] is calculated from Eq.2.17
- ISI [sec^{-1}] is calculated from Eq.2.18
- CO [l/min] is calculated from Eq.2.6.
- BSA [m²] is calculated from Eq.2.2a.
- CI [l/min/m²] from Eq.2.2.
- SI [ml/beat/m²] from Eq.2.7.
- EF estimate [%] is alclculated from Eq.2.17

Explanation of VEPT$_{gender}$:

The Metropolitan Life Insurance Company 1983 tables contain the following information for Mean Ideal Weight (W) [kg] as a function of Height (H) [cm] for both genders:

$W_{Ideal\ Male} = (0.524\ H) - 16.58$ [kg] [Eq.2.21]
$W_{Ideal\ Female} = (0.524\ H) - 26.58$ [kg] [Eq.2.22]

Actual VEPT$_{gender}$ (volume of the electrically participating intrathoracic tissue) is then calculated from Sramek's Equation$^{(11,12)}$ [Eq.2.18] with Bernstein's modification of VEPT by a ratio of patient's actual-to-ideal weight$^{(13)}$:

$VEPT_{gender} = [(0.17H)^3/4.25] \times \{1+0.65[(W/W_{ideal\ gender})-1]\}$ [Eq.2.23]

TEB is a noninvasive counterpart to TD, with no known mortalities and morbidities attributable to the technology. Its clinical accuracy is similar to TD - about ± 20%.

The major difference between these two techniques is in principle of data acquisition: TD displays the mean value of CO over the dilution period (about 12 heartbeats), from which the mean value of SV over the same time period can be calculated. In contrast, TEB determines new SV and CO for every heartbeat. As such, the accuracy of both TD and TEB measured blood flow data is sensitive to severe dysrhythmias and/or motion artifacts, during which the data cannot be acquired and displayed.

The limitations of TEB acquired EF relate to disorders affecting the systolic time intervals, such as the left bundle branch block.

When two techniques for measurement of a physiologic parameter, such as measurement of CO by TD and TEB, are compared to each other, different comparison methods can be utilized. The task usually is to prove or disprove the **clinical agreement** between the two techniques.

The **correlation coefficient may not be used** in this case, since the correlation coefficient method requires that one of the two techniques is an absolutely accurate calibration standard. This is true neither for TD nor for TEB.

Bland/Altman[16], however, described a **correct statistical method** for clinical comparison of two techniques, each having its own range of inaccuracy. This method utilizes graphical plots of comparison points of arithmetic average of both parameters vs. their difference.

Fig.2.8 contains one of published comparisons of TD vs. TEB utilizing the Bland/Altman's method in 100 catheterized patients:

Simultaneous comparisons (each point represents a mean value of 3 measurements) of [(CO$_{TEB}$+CO$_{TD}$)/2] are plotted against [CO_TEB - CO_TD]. This study showed a statistical bias of –0.35 l/min/m², and a reasonably good clinical agreement (a significant majority of the points are within ±20% accuracy band).

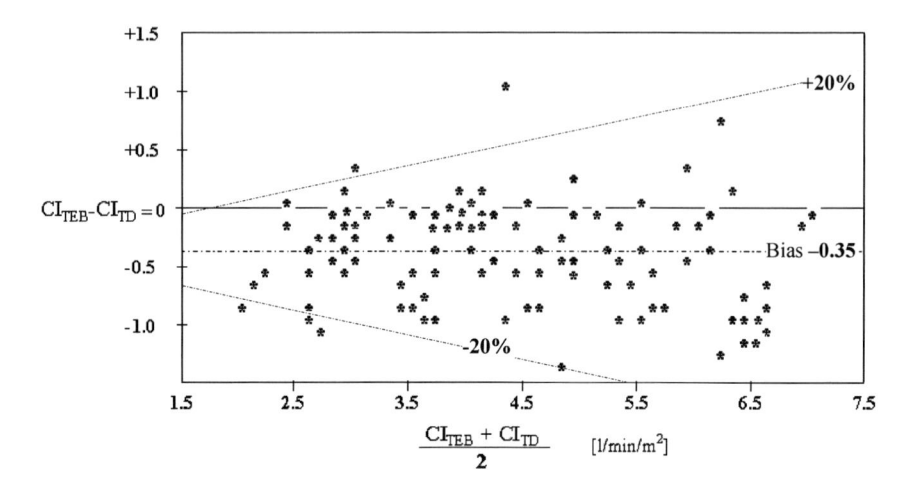

Fig.2.8: Simultaneous CI by TEB and TD (54 men and 46 women, age 20-85 years; mean of 3 measurements). From Arrazola FV: Cardiac Index by TEB and TD: A longitudinal study in 100 patients. Proceedings 4th IHS Int'l Conference on Hemodynamics, Acapulco, Mexico, 1998

Summary:

Braunwald has been right: CO **is** the ultimate expression of cardiovascular performance. As such, its adequacy as a perfusion modulator has to be determined both in inpatients and outpatients. An adequate CO corresponds to adequate O_2 delivery, and, adequate O_2 delivery to all organs equates to cardiovascular health.

TEB is starting to play an important role in CO acquisition: Since it is a noninvasive, continuous and low cost technology with cardiodynamic data available in several minutes after attaching a patient and in any environment, it opens a door to determination of CO in every single patient. This will allow the most significant change within the cardiovascular medicine to take place – a change of health care philosophy from **reactive** (clinical response to a cardiovascular disorder only when it demonstrates itself or is diagnosed) to **proactive** (i.e., maintenance of cardiovascular health).

3. Oxygen Transport: O_2 Delivery and O_2 Consumption

In Chapter 2, we have discussed the role of Cardiac Index (CI) as the only dynamic modulator of oxygen transport, namely **Global O_2 Delivery Index (DO_2I)**, defined as:

$$DO_2I = CI \times 10\ Hgb \times SaO_2 \times 1.34 \qquad [Eq.2.4]$$

Normal values of components of Eq.2.4 for supine, resting adults are:
CI = 3.5 l/min/m² ± 20%
Hgb = 12-16 g/dl females
      14-18 g/dl males
$SaO_2 \geq 94\%$ [3], resulting in
DO_2I = 660 ml/min/m²

Also discussed was the relationship between the value of CI and DO_2I and survival in surgical patients (Eq.2.10 and Eq.2.13).

An interesting aspect of measurement of DO_2I is that now it can be performed continuously and **noninvasively** (CI by TEB and SaO_2 as SpO_2 by Pulse Oximetry). The condition is that Hgb, obtained in the blood laboratory from samples of blood, is updated as frequently as the expected changes of Hgb are taking place. These faster changes of Hgb happen during hemodilution in surgery or during a subsequent transfusion. Otherwise, Hgb is a stable, unchanging parameter and one measurement of Hgb satisfies the condition for a continuous, noninvasive monitoring DO_2I.

However, the process of O_2 transport does not end by delivering O_2 toward body tissues. The tissues have to **extract** O_2 at the cellular level for their metabolic function. As a result of O_2 extraction process, venous blood, returning to the right heart is partially deprived of O_2 and the **Global O_2 Consumption (VO_2I)** is calculated from arterio-venous O_2 saturation difference:

$VO_2I = CI \times 10\, Hgb \times (SaO_2 - SvO_2) \times 1.34$ [Eq.3.1]

where:
SaO_2 is Saturation of O_2 in Arterial Blood [%]
SvO_2 is Saturation of O_2 in Mixed Venous Blood [%] – see explanation below

Normal values of components of Eq.3.1 for supine, resting adults are:
CI = 3.5 l/min/m² ± 20%
Hgb = 12-16 g/dl females
       14-18 g/dl males
SaO_2 = 94-100%[3],
$SvO_2 \cong$ 74-83%[3], resulting in
$VO_2I \cong$ 105-170 ml/min/m²

Since the venous blood returns to the right heart from two separate pathways (superior vena cava and inferior vena cava), VO_2I has to be calculated from the **Saturation of O_2 in Mixed Venous Blood (SvO_2)**; i.e., after both components of the returning venous blood are adequately mixed together. The samples of mixed venous blood can be taken from the pulmonary artery through a corresponding port of the thermodilution catheter, or measured continuously by a special catheter with a blood O_2 saturation sensor located at its tip, which is then placed in the pulmonary artery.

How important is the knowledge of VO_2I in clinical practice? VO_2I is, definitely, the ultimate descriptor of the end-result of the O_2 transport process.

Comments to VO_2I:
- Acquisition of VO_2I can be done only **invasively.**
- If the value of VO_2I is available, it can be compared to norms described in notes to Eq.3.1. and thus confirm adequate or inadequate global O_2 transport conditions.
- Since VO_2I is a **global** O_2 consumption, it cannot identify adequacy and inadequacy of O_2 consumption by individual organs.
- An autonomous increase in O_2 extraction is the last line of defense in a patient's fight for survival. O_2 extraction increases when hemodynamic and perfusion modula-

tion fails to produce adequate DO_2I (reasons: hypovolemia and/or hypoinotropy and/or vasoconstriction and/or hypochronotropy). As of today, there is no known therapeutic process, which could allow the clinician to alter/augment the O_2 extraction…

The therapeutic management of DO_2I is, therefore, a much more clinician-friendly task. As already mentioned, assessment and monitoring DO_2I can be performed noninvasively. Increasing the amount of O_2 to all organs to adequate level (do not forget normal and postoperative goals, described in previous chapter) usually resolves the O_2 deficiency. The exception is a regional inability of individual organs to extract O_2, which exceeds the scope of this book.

There are several therapies, which can augment DO_2I, when needed:

- **Hemodynamic modulation:**
  Volume expansion - with documented hypovolemia

  Positive inotropic support - with documented hypoinotropy

  Afterload reduction - with documented vasoconstriction

- **Perfusion flow modulation:**
  Positive chronotropic therapy - with documented hypochronotropy

- **Blood transfusion**
  with documented hemodilution

These hemodynamic and perfusion flow therapeutic features will be discussed in the following chapter.

4. Hemodynamic Modulation: Per-minute or Per-beat?

4.1. Concepts of Per-minute Hemodynamics

Though a continuous CI by TD catheter is now available, the concepts of hemodynamics and cardiovascular physiology taught at medical schools for the last 30+ years, were conceived and structured around the initial capabilities of TD catheter, that could measure CI and PAOP intermittently, and CVP continuously.

These concepts can be formulated the following way: A patient, who is supine and resting has his oxygen demand at a steady state (unchanging) level. CI, therefore (Eq.2.4), has to be at a steady-state level as well. Ergo, intermittent measurements of CI are satisfactory and only long-term variations of CI are clinically significant. The intermittently measured CI, MAP, PAOP and CVP are subsequently used for calculations of SVRI (afterload), LCWI (Left Cardiac Work Index) and DO_2I, while volemia can be inferred from PAOP. All these parameters then become inputs for therapeutic decisions.

Since the significant global blood flow in current cardiovascular physiology is the CI [l/min/m²], which has a **per-minute physical dimension**, let's call in the following discussion these concepts of hemodynamics **"per-minute" hemodynamics**.

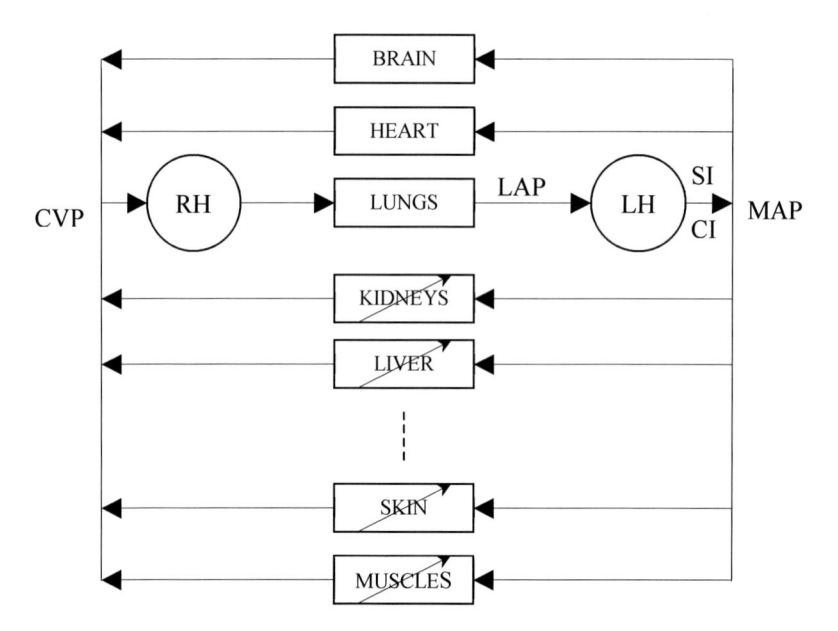

Fig.4.1.1: Schematic diagram of circulatory system as it relates to systemic hemodynamics. Left Heart (LH) delivers SI (blood flow/beat) and CI (blood flow/minute) while creating MAP. Blood pressure drops across the systemic vasculature (different systemic organs marked as such; organs with variable resistance are marked with arrows) to Central Venous Pressure (CVP). The pressure drop across the systemic vasculature is [MAP-CVP]. Blood flowing from the lungs enters the left atrium at the Left Atrial Pressure (LAP). LH elevates the blood pressure from LAP to MAP. LH pressure contribution is [MAP-LAP]. Note: LAP ≅ (PAOP-2)[3]

"Per-minute" hemodynamics concentrates on the following systemic hemodynamic parameters for assessment of a patient's systemic hemodynamics: MAP, PAOP, CI and CVP. Fig.4.1.1 identifies their locations within the systemic circulation.

Please note that PAOP is sometimes referred to as the "wedge" pressure, dating to times before the occlusive balloon on thermodilution catheter was invented and a stiff catheter had to be literally wedged into the pulmonary artery; under this occluded condition, the lungs vasculature becomes a catheter's fluid column extension, allowing to measure the filling pressure of the left heart.

"Per-minute" hemodynamics recognizes the following systemic hemodynamic modulators:

- Preload, defined as the forces of returning blood (from the lungs) stretching myocardial fibers of the left heart, thus storing energy in them during diastole
- Contractility, defined as the forces by which the stretched myocardial fibers contract (shorten) in time during systole
- Afterload, defined as the resistive forces of the systemic vasculature the pump (left ventricle) has to overcome to deliver blood into the systemic vasculature.
- Chronotropic modulation by HR, converting SI (a global blood flow per-beat) into the "hemodynamically significant" CI.

Preload

In **"per-minute" invasive hemodynamics**, preload is synonymous with PAOP: As the **filling pressure** of blood flowing from the lungs increases, the atrial and ventricular walls distend, thus increasing the volume of blood within these chambers, i.e., increasing the **preload.** Normal preload equals to normal PAOP[3] = 6-15 Torr (mean 9 Torr).

This concept is deeply ingrained in minds of physicians, since this is the way it can be measured and also is taught. A special capability of the thermodilution catheter to measure PAOP just further underlined this myth. Even the Frank-Starling Law, the way it is explained and formulated, is defined as a volume-pressure relationship.

Please note a simple fact from both mechanical and biological systems: It is always easier to measure the pressure than the flow.

The **physical and physiological facts** of preload, however, are different. Preload is not related to filling blood pressure but to **blood volume**. Blood flowing from the lungs has a kinetic energy in the form of **inertia**. This kinetic energy is the preload force, which stretches the left atrial wall fibers and, subsequently, the ventricular wall fibers, thus storing energy in them. In the process of filling the atrium, **a pressure** (LAP) develops, **not as a cause** but as **a consequence** of **blood inflow** and chamber **compliance**. The unknown wall compliance is the Achilles heel of reliance on pressures to assess blood volume: With a compliant ventricular wall of a young patient, the patient can be volume overloaded with PAOP = 14 Torr (still considered a normal value) and, in contrast, an old patient with a stiff ventricle, can be profoundly volume depleted with the same PAOP = 14 Torr.

In **"per-minute" noninvasive hemodynamics**, preload is synonymous with the **End-Diastolic Index (EDI)** [ml/m^2] – the BSA-indexed volume of blood accumulated in the left ventricle at the end of the diastolic filling phase.

Since we describe the heart as a mechanical, pulsatile blood flow generator (pulsatile pump), we have to consider its related blood volume transfer properties. While discussing **EDI**, we should mention the pump's emptying capability, described by **Ejection Fraction (EF)**, defined as

$$\mathbf{EF = SI/EDI \times 100} \ [\%] \qquad [Eq.4.1]$$

EF is typically classified into four ranges:
High   EF > 65%
Normal 50% < EF < 65%
Low   35% < EF < 50%
Poor   EF < 35%

When **EF** is measured and **SI** is known, **EDI** (hence the preload) can be calculated as

$$\mathbf{EDI = SI/EF \times 100} \ [ml/m^2] \qquad [Eq.4.1a]$$

Normal values of input parameters for adults are:
SI$_{normal}$ = 47 ml/m^2 ± 34% (Eq.2.7)

$EF_{normal} = 57.5\% \pm 15\%$ (Eq.4.1)
resulting in $EDI_{normal} = 82$ ml/m$^2 \pm 49\%$

In view of normal ranges of SI ($\pm$ 34%) and EF ($\pm$ 15%), the resulting normal range of EDI becomes very broad ($\pm$ 49%), making it a very imprecise means for assessment of preload.

EF is calculated from images of the left ventricle, obtained by X-ray or ultrasound techniques, which are **slow** and **expensive** processes. These images are either single plane or two-dimensional images of End-Diastolic and End-Systolic Volumes. Since the ventricle is not a perfect rotational object (neither at the end of diastole nor at the end of systole), volumes calculated from these images exhibit a limited accuracy. In addition, in view of the facts discussed in Chapter 4.2 (see Fig.4.2.1), the left ventricle never has the same size even in two consecutive heartbeats, adding to inaccuracy of already broad ($\pm$ 49%) normal range of EF determinations obtained by imaging techniques.

Note that a noninvasive estimate of EF can be obtained continuously by TEB (Eq.2.19) from the Systolic Time Intervals[15].

Notes to EF measurements:

The protagonists of "per-minute" hemodynamics herald EF as one of the most important noninvasively obtained parameters describing the left ventricular performance.

Is it true?

EF describes the pumps emptying capability, not directly related to the pump's primary function – supply of oxygen to tissues and organs. It is probably true that a heart with higher EF has a better reserve under physical load conditions. On the other hand, it is also known that marathon runners (i.e., top athletes) have a very low EF shortly after finishing the race.

In absence of complete hemodynamic assessment, discussed in the following chapters, knowledge of EF may shed some light on the status of the cardiovascular system, when compared to poor hemodynamic informational values of current HR and S/D pressure measurements. However, since there is no simple therapy to improve a low EF, the true perceived value of EF might be in allowing calculation of EDI, thus preload.

Contractility

Contractility is the force by which the myocardial fibers, with energy stored in them during the ventricular filling (stretched during diastole), shorten in time during systole. More stretched fibers shorten with a higher force (Frank-Starling Law). There also are known pharmacological effects of inotropes on contractility: positive inotropes increase it, negative inotropes decrease it, though many physicians consider contractility and inotropy to be synonymous.

In "per-minute" hemodynamics, contractility is not routinely measured. A relative assessment of contractility can be performed with ultrasound, though no norms for its measurement have been adopted.

Afterload

"Per-minute" hemodynamics assesses the primary component of afterload through the **Systemic Vascular Resistance Index (SVRI)**, defined as

$SVRI = 80 \times (MAP-CVP)/CI$ [dyn.sec.cm^{-5}.m^2] [Eq.4.2]

Normal values of the parameters for adults are[3]:
MAP = 85 Torr
CVP = 4 Torr
CI = 3.5 l/min/m^2
resulting in normal (ideal) value of SVRI = 1851 dyn.sec.cm^{-5}.m^2

The secondary component of afterload is blood viscosity, related to Hgb; however, with the exception of extreme hemodilution or hemoconcentration, it does not have to be considered in clinical decisions affecting afterload.

We will not discuss here the use of an unindexed counterpart to SVRI – the **Systemic Vascular Resistance (SVR)** – defined as

$SVR = 80 \times (MAP-PAOP)/CO$ [dyn.sec.cm^{-5}] [Eq.4.2a]

Though **SVR** is still popular with some physicians, it **represents** a totally **incorrect assessment of afterload**, leading to its complete misdiagnoses and resulting in an incorrect afterload modification therapy. The reasons have been discussed in Chapter 2: Neither CO nor SVR exhibit a normal range. The calculated SVR value, therefore, just becomes a calculated number, useless for any therapeutic decisions.

Chronotropy

In addition to augmentation of SI (see Fig.2.2 and related discussion), chronotropic compensation by HR is responsible for augmentation of CI in response to an increased oxygen demand. Positive chronotropes increase HR, while negative chronotropes decrease it. In "per-minute" hemodynamics, the absolute value of HR becomes the measure of chronotropy: Bradycardia = hypochronotropy; tachycardia = hyperchronotropy (we will discuss in the following chapters how incorrect this assessment of chronotropy is).

Left Cardiac Work Index

Left Cardiac Work Index (LCWI) describes the amount of physical work the left heart expends in one minute to pump (energize) the blood arriving from the lungs at LAP (Left Atrial Pressure) level to a higher, MAP pressure level – see Fig.4.1.1.

LCWI is a classical "per-minute" component, defined as[5]

LCWI = 0.0144 (MAP-LAP) x CI   [kg.m/m²]   [Eq.4.3]

Normal values of the parameters for adults are[3]:
MAP = 85 Torr
LAP = 7 Torr
CI = 3.5 l/min/m²
resulting in $LCWI_{normal}$ = 3.93 kg.m/m²

From a physical viewpoint, LCWI represents the work the left heart expends every minute; its ideal value is equivalent of lifting 3.93 kg to a height of 1 m per every m² of BSA.

Physiologically, LCWI parallels the **"per-minute" myocardial oxygen consumption.**

In "per-minute" hemodynamics, the sequence of hemodynamic and oxygen delivery dynamics modulation is perceived the following way:

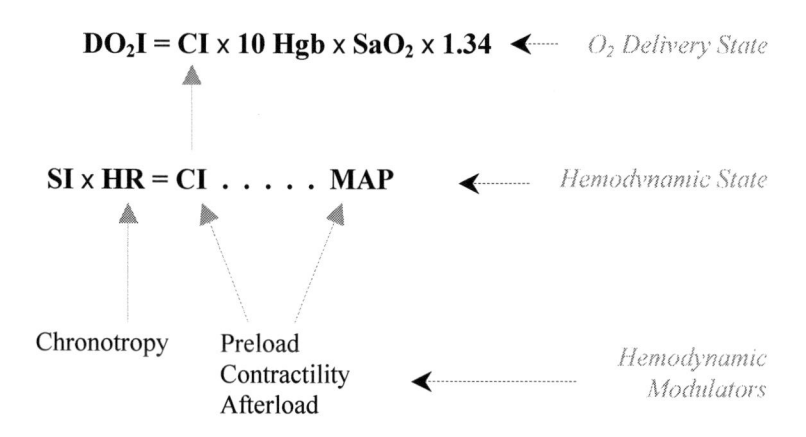

$$DO_2I = CI \times 10\, Hgb \times SaO_2 \times 1.34 \quad \longleftarrow \quad O_2\ Delivery\ State$$

$$SI \times HR = CI\ .\ .\ .\ .\ .\ MAP \quad \longleftarrow \quad Hemodynamic\ State$$

Chronotropy   Preload
               Contractility $\longleftarrow$ *Hemodynamic Modulators*
               Afterload

Fig.4.1.2: Schematic diagram of hemodynamics and oxygen delivery dynamics and their modulation pathways, as perceived by "per-minute" hemodynamics. The therapy usually concentrates on treating either CI or MAP (or S/D measured blood pressures).

Hemodynamic Management under "Per-minute" Hemodynamics

Fig.4.1.2 above depicts the modulating pathways applicable to "per-minute" hemodynamics. Please note that the diagnosed global blood flow deviations (CI) from its established norms are, typically, treated separately from diagnosed blood pressure deviations (MAP) from its established norms.

In "per-minute" hemodynamics the major indicators activating the therapeutic process depend on the type of patient and on detected deviation either in blood pressure or in blood flow from their established norms:

- In **outpatients,** the therapeutic decisions related to hemodynamics are mostly derived from Systolic/Diastolic arterial blood pressure measurement.

    If **hypertension** is detected
    (S $\geq$ 140 Torr, or D $\geq$ 90 Torr), administer:

    (a) diuretics, and/or
    (b) beta blockers, and/or
    (c) calcium channel blockers, and/or
    (d) ACE inhibitors

    NIH (National Institute of Health)[19] and drug manufacturers provide guidelines for selection of antihypertensive drug(s). The current hemodynamic goal is to reduce the blood pressure to a normotensive level. Last NIH Report[19], covering the period 1991-94, lists the following outcome-related US numbers: 53.6% of hypertensives were treated, out of which 27.4% had their hypertension controlled (i.e., 72.6% of treated hypertensives remained hypertensive in spite of taking antihypertensive medications).

- **In inpatients**, which are **not catheterized**, the therapeutic decisions related to hemodynamics essentially follow the methodology and guidelines for outpatients, listed above.

    In inpatients with TD catheters (< 2% of inpatients), the measurements and therapeutic decisions related to hemodynamics represent a fairly complex matrix of measurements and therapeutic responses. Ultimately, they can be narrowed down to the following processes:

(a) **Measurement of PAOP:**
Measured PAOP is compared to its normal range of $6 < PAOP < 16$ Torr[3]:

Therapy:
When PAOP < 6 Torr, implying hypovolemia, start volume expansion;
when PAOP > 16 Torr, implying hypervolemia, administer volume reduction (diureses).

(b) **Measurement of CI in nonsurgical patients:**
CI is compared to the normal range[3] of $2.8 < CI < 4.2$ l/min/m².

Therapy:
When CI < 2.5 l/min/m² and PAOP < 6 Torr (implying a low flow state with contribution of hypovolemia) start immediately volume expansion + positive inotropic therapy + afterload reduction (vasodilatation). Goal is CI = 3.5 l/min/m²

(c) **Measurement of CI in patients after a major surgery**[3]:
CI is compared to the normal range of $3.6 < CI < 5.4$ l/min/m²

(Please note that this Postoperative Therapeutic Goal is used only in some institutions familiar with the methodology described by Shoemaker et al[3])

Therapy:
Same as in (b), however, with a different normal range of
$3.6 < CI < 5.4$ l/min/m²; goal is CI = 4.5 l/min/m².

This "blanket CI augmentation therapy" (volume expansion + positive inotropic therapy + afterload reduction) does not attempt to correct the **actual** deficiencies in hemodynamic modulators, i.e., determined levels of hypovolemia, hypoinotropy and vasoconstriction. Its goal is just a rapid augmentation of CI.

Notes to the Postoperative Therapeutic Goal for Adult Patients with Major Surgery:

More than 24 million major surgical operations are performed annually in the US with an estimated annual mortality of over 400,000[5]. The postoperative therapeutic goal for surgical survivors (see Chapter 2 for detailed discussion) addresses one potential way of reducing postoperative mortalities.

In following chapters, we will discuss a more effective way of further reducing mortalities of major surgical operations, improving management of hypertension and congestive heart failure and allowing the physicians to manage and maintain their in- and outpatients in a desired hemodynamic state.

4.2. Concepts of "Per-beat" Hemodynamics

A minute, used in "per-minute" hemodynamics, is a man-invented measure of time, totally unrelated to the basic clock of the cardiovascular system, which is **one heartbeat**.

A convention to name CO as a blood flow the heart pumps in one minute can probably be traced to a known fact that, at rest, the normal blood volume is turned over by heart approximately once every minute.

However, imagine, that we had adopted in the past a convention to name CO not as blood flow/minute, but blood flow/hour, blood flow/day... You can see from this example that so more we expand the averaging time period for blood flow, so less visible the short-term blood flow variations become. If we would go to an ultimate extreme and adopt CO to be blood flow/life, we would not have to measure this parameter. The measured CO would be normal in all subjects, because the periods of low-flow states, linked to mortalities in major surgical operations, would not be visible at all.

Fig. 4.2.1 describes "per-beat" hemodynamic measurements recorded by a scientist studying respiratory patterns and their effects on hemodynamics of a resting, reclining, healthy normal adult male (supine or reclining posture is a typical posture, in which the majority of hemodynamic measurements are performed). This **normal, resting subject** must have his oxygen demand at a steady state level, resulting in DO_2I to be at a steady state. Under these conditions, CI should, therefore, be at a steady state level as well (Eq.2.4). If CI is at a steady state, and there are no other stimuli to affect hemodynamics, then the recordings of HR and SI (Eq.2.6) in Fig.4.2.1 should be straight horizontal lines. And, if under these steady state conditions the vascular tone (SVRI – see Eq.4.2) is unchanging, then the MAP recording should be a straight horizontal line as well.

However, as Fig.4.2.1 shows, all three measured parameters exhibit profound beat-by-beat variations:
MAP varies ± 7.5% from its mean value of 94.5 Torr,
SI varies ± 31% from its mean value of 35.5 ml/beat/m^2,
HR varies ± 20% from its mean value of 70 beats/min.

Since this is not a patient with any known hemodynamic abnormality, the only conclusion we can reach is that **even under steady-state oxygen demand,** the cardiovascular system keeps on adjusting itself continuously into **a new hemodynamic state** (paired values of blood flow and blood pressure) **for every heartbeat** and the "per-minute" concepts of hemodynamics are fundamentally flawed.

Let's identify the causes and the consequences of these rapid per-beat variations:

As discussed in detail in Chapter 2, the leading hemodynamic component (the cause) is the **blood flow**, in this case it is the global blood flow per-beat - the **SI.**

You can clearly see in Fig.4.2.1 a steady state background mean level of SI ≅ 35.5 ml/beat/m^2, responding on a long-term basis to the steady-state O_2 demand. However, superimposed on this steady-state level are other SI variations:

There are the beat-by-beat SI variations caused by respiration, which should be expected: Inspiration, with negative intrathoracic pressure, increases preload, thus the SI value, while expiration, with positive intrathoracic pressure, decreases it. These respiratory variations, having frequency of about ¼ of heart rate frequency and amplitude of about ± 1-2 ml/beat/m^2, are clearly visible in Fig. 4.2.1.

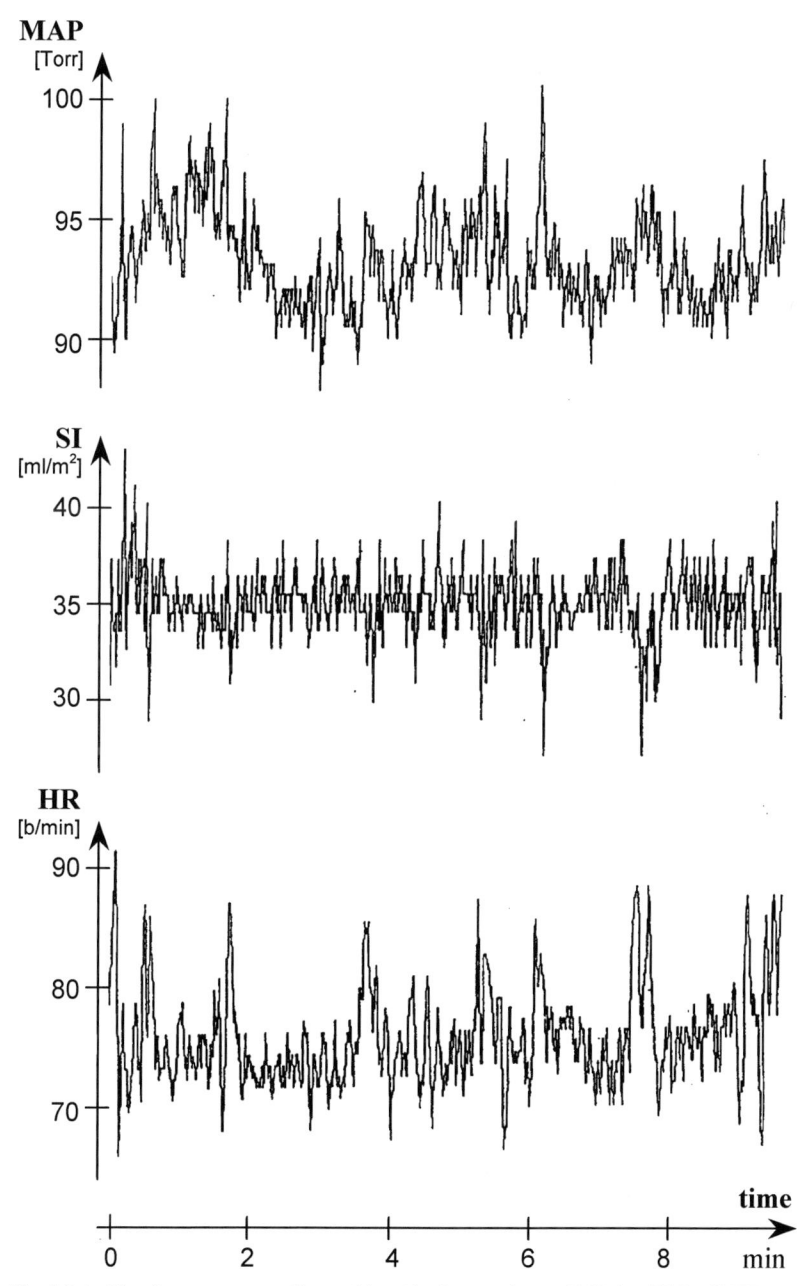

Fig.4.2.1: Simultaneous recordings of beat-by-beat values of HR (by ECG of TEB System), SI (by TEB System) and MAP (by FinaPress) over a 10-minute period in a reclining, resting adult male. Courtesy David Shannahoff-Khalsa, The Research Group for Mind-Body Dynamics, Institute for Nonlinear Science, University of California San Diego, California

Striking, though, are the large SI excursions, mostly negative and random in appearance, taking place about every 20-150 seconds. These are the Mayer waves[22], representing the central nervous system's reset signals to compensate for inability of cardiovascular biofeedbacks to have a DC transfer component within the biofeedback loop.

During the Mayer waves, the SI decreases momentarily by 20-30% from its mean value, determined by the oxygen demand. This blood flow decrease is, however, immediately recognized. The hemodynamic response to a decreased SI is a chronotropic compensatory increase in HR, which purpose is to maintain CI, therefore DO_2I, at a level in which O_2 demand and supply are in equilibrium. You can clearly see that every Mayer wave-caused SI decrease is matched by a corresponding increase in HR.

One additional conclusion from Fig.4.2.1 can be reached:

If the systemic vascular resistance (SVRI in "per-minute" hemodynamics) would be only slowly (per-minute) responding to its task to distribute the available blood flow among all organs, then the per-beat MAP recording would have to be an image of SI (blood pressure would copy the blood flow). However, as you can see from Fig.4.2.1, **MAP is not an image of SI**, leading to a conclusion, that the beat-by-beat variations of SI are accompanied by **independent, beat-by-beat variations of vascular resistance**.

The **SVRI** (Eq.4.2), currently used in "per-minute" hemodynamics as a parameter for assessment of afterload, is, therefore, **flawed**. If the vasculature adjusts the caliber of arterioles at the input to each organ (a new vascular resistance value) for every heartbeat, then the correct component for assessment of afterload must be its per-beat parameter - the **Stroke Systemic Vascular Resistance Index, SSVRI,** defined as

$$SSVRI = 80 \, (MAP - CVP)/SI \quad [dyn.sec.cm^{-5}.m^2] \quad [Eq.4.4]$$

Ideal values for supine, resting adults are[3]:
MAP_{ideal} = 85 Torr
CVP_{ideal} = 4 Torr
SI_{ideal} = 47 ml/m²
resulting in an ideal value of $SSVRI_{ideal}$ = 137.8 dyn.sec.cm⁻⁵.m²

SVRI is not only physiologically incorrect but its use can lead to misdiagnoses and, subsequently, have devastating clinical consequences through an incorrectly selected therapy. Let's explain this point on an example listed in Table 4.1:

	SI	CI	HR	MAP	CVP	SVRI	SSVRI
Ideal Patient[3]	47	3.5	74.5	85	4	1851	137.8
Hemodynamically Compromised Patient	35	3.5	100	85	4	1851	185 (+34%)

Table 4.1: This table contains hemodynamic data of two patients: An ideal patient, and a patient, who is in a lower-than-normal flow state (SI=35), normotensive (MAP=85), however, due to a correct chronotropic compensation by HR (HR=100), still has a normal perfusion blood flow (CI=3.5). Values of SVRI and SSVRI were calculated from Eq.4.2 and Eq.4.4.

The first row in Table 4.1 is for an ideal patient[3], resulting in values of SVRI = 1851 dyn.sec.cm⁻⁵.m² and SSVRI = 137.8 dyn.sec.cm⁻⁵.m². Both of these values can be considered to be "normal" or "ideal" values for supine resting adults.

The second row contains data of another patient whose SI = 35 ml/m² (a decreased global blood flow/beat by 34% from its normal value of 47 ml/m²), however, due to correct chronotropic compensation by HR = 100 beats/min, his CI = 3.5 l/min/m², which is still an ideal CI value.

Should the clinician educated in "per-minute" hemodynamics decide to therapeutically treat the low SI value in the second patient, he would eliminate any afterload therapy as a legitimate choice, since the SVRI, i.e., the measure of afterload, is at an ideal level, and would concentrate on therapeutic management of two remaining modulators: volume expansion and/or positive inotropic therapy. To his surprise, the patient's response to the selected therapy would be a temporary increase of SI, however, accompanied by an increase in arterial blood pressure (hypertension).

When we look at the value of **SSVRI** of the second patient, we can see that his **"per-beat" afterload** is +34% higher than the ideal SSVRI value – the patient is actually 34% **vasoconstricted**, a fact hidden by SVRI; CI, used in SVRI calculation, already includes the chronotropic compensation by HR.

Since the chronotropic compensation by HR is the second from the last line of defenses of cardiovascular system to achieve adequate oxygen delivery even with hemodynamic decompensation (an increased oxygen extraction at the tissue level being the last one), the majority of hemodynamically compromised patients a clinician will see will be the patients with low SI, increased HR, close-to-normal CI and, therefore, incorrectly derived value of afterload if SVRI is used for its assessment.

From the preceding discussion related to Fig.4.2.1 and derived conclusions, we can redraw the functional schematic diagram of hemodynamics as follows:

$$DO_2I = CI \times 10\, Hgb \times SaO_2 \times 1.34 \quad \longleftarrow \quad \textit{O}_2 \textit{ Delivery}$$

$$CI = SI \times HR \quad \longleftarrow \quad \textit{Perfusion Blood Flow}$$

Chronotropy

$$SI \quad @ \quad MAP \quad \longleftarrow \quad \textit{Hemodynamic State}$$

Hemodynamic Modulators:
Intravascular Volume
← *Contractility* ←
Inotropy
← *Vasoactivity*

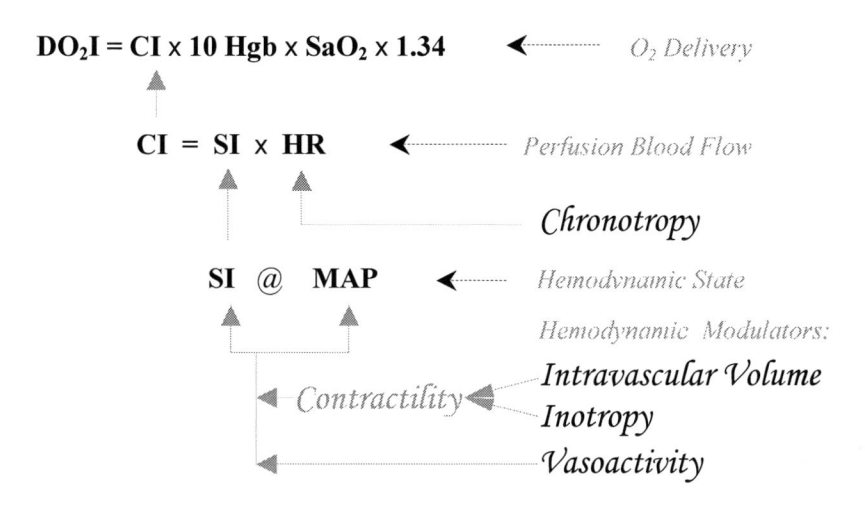

Fig.4.2.2: Schematic diagram of hemodynamic, perfusion blood flow and oxygen delivery modulation, as understood under "per-beat" hemodynamics. Solid arrows show the direction of hemodynamic modulation: Three hemodynamic modulators (intravascular volume, inotropy and vasoactivity) are responsible for a Hemodynamic State, defined as a new pair of SI and MAP, formed for every heartbeat. Chronotropy then modulates the hemodynamically formed SI value by HR. Chronotropic modulation is attempting to achieve such a level in Perfusion Blood Flow (CI) as to accomplish adequate O_2 Delivery.

The sequence of hemodynamic, perfusion flow and O_2 delivery modulation, therefore, can be described as follows:

- The levels of three hemodynamic modulators (intravascular volume, inotropy and vasoactivity), each changing its status in **multivectorial** fashion for every heartbeat, are responsible for the **hemodynamic state**, defined as paired values of SI & MAP.
- A new hemodynamic state is formed for every heartbeat.

- Hemodynamically significant global blood flow is **SI**, hemodynamically significant blood pressure is **MAP**.

- Depending on (1) a level of **SI** formed by hemodynamic modulation, and (2) status of **Hgb** and **SaO₂** at O_2 delivery level, chronotropic modulation by **HR** attempts to establish an adequate level of **perfusion blood flow** - the **CI** – as to produce **normal level** of **DO₂I**.

- **CI** thus is the true dynamic **perfusion blood flow** parameter, responding both to the available input level of **SI** and to required output level of **DO₂I**.

As the per-beat counterpart to SVRI is the SSVRI, the per-beat counterpart to LCWI (Eq.4.3) is the **Left Stroke Work Index, LSWI,** defined as

$$\text{LSWI} = 0.0144 \, (\text{MAP} - \text{LAP}) \times \text{SI} \quad [\text{g.m/m}^2] \quad [\text{Eq.4.5}]$$

Ideal values for supine, resting adults are[3]:
MAP_{ideal} = 85 Torr
LAP_{ideal} = 7 Torr
SI_{ideal} = 47 ml/m²,
resulting in LSWI_{ideal} = 52.8 g.m/m²

LSWI represents the mean value of physical work the left heart expends over one heart beat interval; the ideal value of 52.8 g.m/m² represents a work needed to lift 52.8 grams by 1 meter per every meter square of BSA. Physiologically, it parallels the **per-beat myocardial oxygen consumption**.

We will discus the hemodynamic significance of LSWI in the following section of this textbook.

4.2.1. Hemodynamic Modulators

4.2.1.1. Preload: Intravascular Volume Modulation

Preload represents the effects of inertial forces of pulmonary venous blood return, stretching the relaxed myocardial fibers during diastole, thus storing mechanical energy in them. Preload is associated with the transformation of kinetic energy of flowing blood during diastolic ventricular filling into the static energy of myocardial fibers' tension. Ventricular compliance, ultimately, determines the magnitude of ventricular filling.

Preload is a **diastolic** phenomenon.

The modulating pathway of preload is a variation of intravascular blood volume available to the pump. Preload modulation thus may be accomplished by:

- Redistribution of intravascular volume with change in posture (a supine position is associated with a higher level of preload in comparison to standing upright due to diminished effects of gravity),
- venoconstriction (mobilization of blood from venous compartment increases preload),
- therapeutic intervention (volume expansion increases preload, diureses decreases it),
- change in ventricular compliance.

Preload (i.e., the intravascular volume level) can attain three distinctive levels:

- **Normovolemia** – normal (adequate) level of active (circulating) blood volume.

- **Hypovolemia** (volume depletion) – infranormal level of active (circulating) blood volume
- **Hypervolemia** (volume overload) – supernormal level of active (circulating) blood volume

All three levels of blood volume listed above (hypo-, normo-, or hypervolemia) are **relative** terms: The same **circulating** blood volume under a different metabolic/circulatory condition can become inadequate, normal or excessive.

4.2.1.2. Myocardial Contractility: Mechanical & Pharmacological Modulation

Myocardial contractility represents the forces associated with the rate of shortening of myocardial fibers in time during the mechanical systole. Mechanical systole is divided into two parts, the isovolumic contraction and the ejection phase. Therefore, we have to develop and understand the concepts of contractility within these two systolic phases. In addition, contractility is an end-result of two separate phenomena, which affect the rate of shortening of myocardial fibers – the physical mechanism (Frank-Starling Law) and a pharmacological mechanism (inotropy).

a) Isovolumic Phase Contractility (see Fig.4.2.3)

In respect to its timing, the isovolumic phase encompasses the Pre-Ejection Period (PEP). PEP starts at the Q-time of the ECG QRS complex and ends at AVO-time (Aortic Valve Opening).

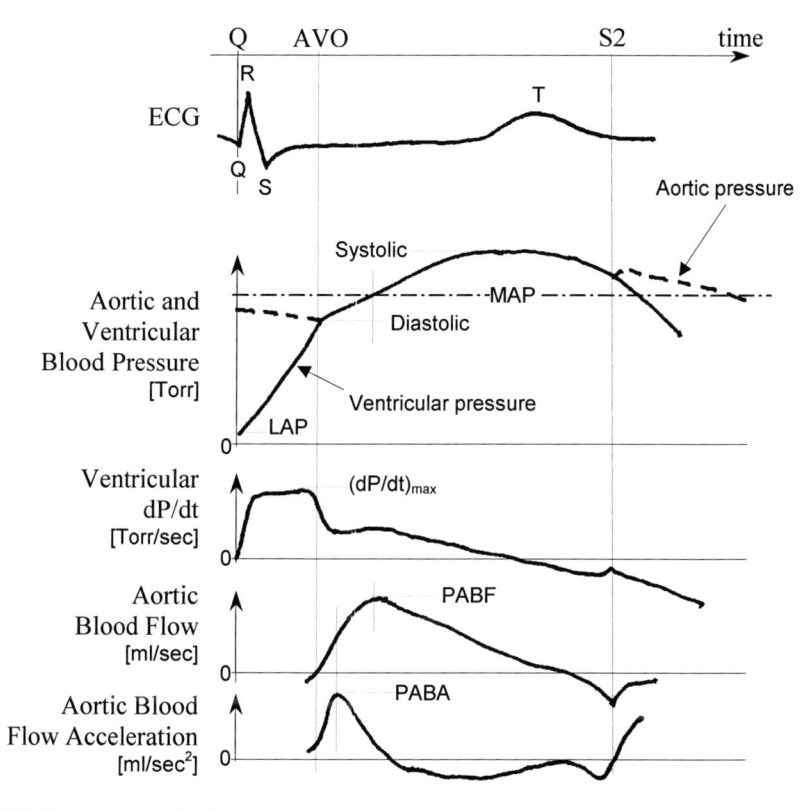

Fig.4.2.3: Relationship of different parameters within the electromechanical systole: The Q-time of ECG QRS complex starts the timing; it ends at the S2 (the second sound), i.e., the closure of aortic valve. AVO = Aortic Valve Opening time is marked. Shown is the relationship between **(a)** ECG, **(b)** ventricular blood pressure (solid line) and aortic blood pressure (dotted line); pressure levels - LAP = Left Atrial Pressure, S = Systolic, D = Diastolic, and MAP are marked, **(c)** ventricular blood pressure rate in time (dP/dt), **(d)** aortic blood flow [PABF = Peak Aortic Blood Flow is marked] and **(e)** aortic blood flow acceleration [PABA = Peak Aortic Blood Flow Acceleration is marked].

At the Q-time, the ventricular pressure is at the LAP level, with a typical value of 7 Torr. As the myocardial fibers start to contract, the left ventricular pressure exhibits a small rise, causing the mitral valve to close. From this moment, the isovolumic contraction, defined as an almost linear and rapid rate of rise of ventricular pressure, takes place. This pressure rise ends when the ventricular pressure incrementally exceeds the Diastolic pressure level and the aortic valve opens at AVO-time.

A typical normal Diastolic pressure in adults is 80 Torr. PEP, therefore, is defined as (Q-AVO) time period.

Contraction of myocardial fibers produces tension along the ventricular wall. Since blood is a noncompressible fluid, the rate of contraction results in a rate of ventricular pressure rise, dP/dt [Torr/sec]. The isovolumic dP/dt, with its maximum rate (dP/dt)$_{max}$, is fairly independent of loading parameters (preload and afterload)[21], and is controlled, essentially, by the inotropic state only. The inotropy/inotropic state is related to the effects of certain pharmacological agents – inotropes (circulating within blood) - on contractility: Positive inotropes increase the contractility, negative inotropes decrease it. (dP/dt)$_{max}$, therefore, becomes a measure of inotropic state. Normal, mean value of (dP/dt)$_{max}$, i.e., **normoinotropy,** is defined as (dP/dt)$_{max} \cong 700$ Torr/sec.

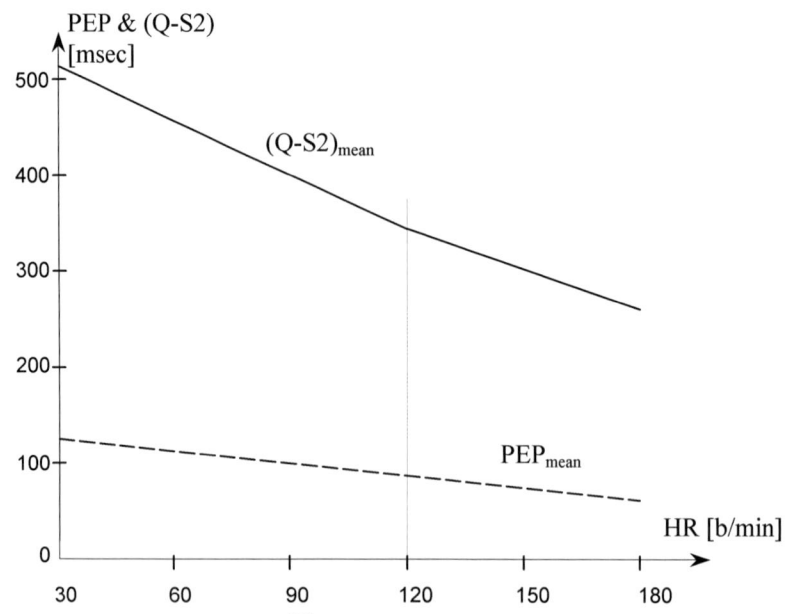

Fig.4.2.4: Systolic Time Intervals[20]: Relationships of mean values of (Q-S2) and PEP in normal adult man as a function of HR. A change of heart function from a variable output volume to constant volume device at HR $\cong$ 120 b/min is visible on (Q-S2)$_{mean}$. Compare to Fig.2.2. The time difference [(Q-S2) – PEP] = VET (Ventricular Ejection Time).

Fig.4.2.4 shows the relationship between PEP and HR. Since PEP decreases slightly with an increasing HR[20], the inotropic state exhibits a slight dependence on chronotropy.

The isovolumic ventricular pressure buildup is proportional to mechanical energy production within the myocardium. Close to 75% of myocardial oxygen is consumed during this phase. Myocardial oxygen consumption is proportional both to absolute value of pressure rise (MAP-LAP) and to its rate dP/dt. The energy, stored in form of pressure buildup, is then released at the AVO time. The instantaneous energy release delivers a mechanical impulse to the stationary ventricular blood (the left ventricular impulse), which produces the initial movement of blood particles toward and into the aortic valve orifice. The left ventricular impulse is converted into the maximum rate of aortic blood flow, i.e., into the **Peak Aortic Blood Flow Acceleration** (PABA) [ml/m^2] – Fig.4.2.3. PABA is firmly based upon theories of fluid dynamics and its derivation is free of assumptions related to heart structure and functions[21].

Since the time of PABA is only about 30 msec after the AVO time[21], only a negligible amount of mechanical energy is wasted in form of heat and its significant portion, accumulated during isovolumic contraction and proportional to ∫dP/dt, is converted into PABA. The PABA value thus correlates very closely to (dP/dt)$_{max}$ and becomes an **alternative measure of inotropic state.**

Though both (dP/dt)$_{max}$ and PABA represent a measure of the inotropic state, there is a major difference between them: (dP/dt)$_{max}$ can be measured only invasively and intermittently via a special catheter, retrograde-inserted through the femoral artery all the way into the left ventricle, with a microchip pressure transducer at its tip – a highly invasive, costly and risky procedure. In contrast, PABA can be measured noninvasively and intermittently by Doppler Ultrasound and noninvasively and continuously by

TEB (see a discussion of TEB in Chapter 2). The TEB measurement of inotropy is called the **Inotropic State Index (ISI)** with a physical dimension $1/\sec^2 = \sec^{-2}$.

Normal levels of ISI according to gender and age are in Table 4.2:

	ISI_{min} [sec^{-2}]	ISI_{ideal} [sec^{-2}]	ISI_{max} [sec^{-2}]
Female young	1.00	1.35	1.70
Female old	0.85	1.20	1.55
Male young	0.85	1.15	1.45
Male old	0.75	1.10	1.30

Table 4.2: Normal values of noninvasive measurement of inotropy via Inotropic State Index (see Eq.2.18 for definition) - Courtesy HEMO SAPIENS® INC. Normal ISI values for young patients are fairly flat till approx. age 55, when they start declining, reaching "old" values at about age 70.

b) Ejection Phase Contractility (see Fig.4.2.3)

The ejection phase contractility encompasses the time period between opening of the aortic valve (AVO-time) and its closure (S2-time in Fig.4.2.3). This period is called the **Ventricular Ejection Time, VET** [sec].

The ejection phase contractility is a superimposed sum of two modulating pathways, mechanical (volume) and pharmacological (inotropy). Fig.4.2.5 explains the relationship between these two pathways.

Fig.4.2.5 describes the Frank-Starling relationship between **Intravascular Volume** and **Ejection Phase Contractility (EPC)**. The variable parameter of this nonlinear relationship is **Inotropy**:

- **Pharmacological Contribution (inotropy):**

Let's assume that the intravascular volume (preload) is at its normal level (marked "Normovolemia") and the inotropic state is also at its normal level (marked "Normoinotropy"). This normal operating point is marked by a little circle. Patient, whose hemodynamics is at this point, will exhibit a "Normal" level of EPC.

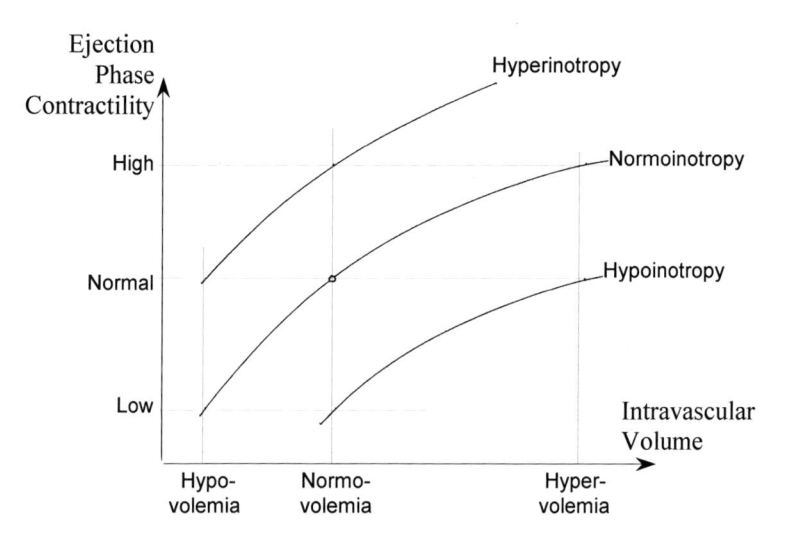

Fig.4.2.5: Frank-Starling Law and Inotropy: Three Frank-Starling curves shown – normoinotropy, hyperinotropy and hypoinotropy. A patient, who is normovolemic and normoinotropic, exhibits normal level of Ejection Phase Contractility (EPC). However, a patient who is hypovolemic can exhibit the same normal level of EPC if given positive inotropes, and, a patient who is volume overloaded (hypervolemic) can also have normal level of EPC if given negative inotropes.

With the presence of positive inotropes (produced by the patient or administered therapeutically), there will be an increase in contractility (an upward shift to a curve marked "Hyperinotropy"), which encompasses both the isovolumic contractility, as discussed above in the corresponding paragraph, and the EPC. In Fig.4.2.5 this increase in inotropy results in an increase in EPC from a level marked "Normal" to a level marked "High." Please note that this increase in EPC took place without any change in preload (intravascular volume). This pharmacologically induced increase in EPC is represented by an upward shift of the entire Frank-Starling curve from "Normoinotropy" to "Hyperinotropy." Obviously, negative inotropes (produced or administered) will reduce EPC from level marked "Normal" to a level marked "Low." Presence of negative inotropes is represented by a shift of the entire Frank-Starling curve downward to a level marked "Hypoinotropy."

- **Mechanical (Frank-Starling) Contribution:**

    Let's assume again that the intravascular volume (preload) is at its normal level (marked "Normovolemia") and the inotropic state is also at its normal level (marked "Normoinotropy"). An increase in intravascular volume from level marked "Normovolemia" to a level marked "Hypervolemia" will result in an increase in EDI and more stretched myocardial fibers at the end of diastole. It will also move the contractility operating point **along** the corresponding normoinotropic Frank-Starling curve right and up. More stretched myocardial fibers shorten with a higher force in the next systole and will result in an increase in EPC from "Normal" to "High." This volume manipulation is performed at a constant inotropic level. Obviously, volume reduction (diuresis) has an opposite effect on EPC, producing a decrease in EPC from "Normal" to "Low."

Shortening myocardial fibers during the ejection phase causes a transfer of part of the ventricular volume into the aorta, i.e., the aortic blood flow (= **SI**).

[The residual blood volume left in the left ventricle at the end of ejection phase is called the End-Systolic Volume (ESV) and is related to EF (see the discussion related to Eq.4.1: EDV = ESV + SV)].

An increase in aortic blood flow produces an increase in aortic blood pressure across the systemic vascular impedance (see Fig.1.1 and Fig.4.2.3). The maximum ejection force takes place at the optimal performance point of systemic hemodynamics: At the time when aortic blood flow reaches its maximum value (PABF), the aortic blood pressure is crossing the MAP value.

4.2.1.3 Afterload: Vasoactivity Modulation

Afterload represents the resistive forces of systemic vasculature, which the left ventricle must overcome in order to deliver the bolus of blood, equivalent to SI, into the systemic vasculature (for every heart beat).

The primary modulating pathway of afterload is a variation of **vasoactivity**, i.e., changing the caliber of sphincters at the input and output of systemic organs, thus producing a change in organ's vascular resistance for every heartbeat. Afterload is also affected by large vessels compliance changes.

The secondary modulating pathway of afterload is a variation in **blood viscosity**, which may be neglected with the exception of profound hemodilution or hemoconcentration.

Afterload, though not totally equivalent to, can be represented by the **SSVRI** (see Eq.4.4). SSVRI represents a parallel sum of all organs' vascular resistances transformed to the output node of the pump (see Fig.4.1.1).

Global vasodilatation represents afterload reduction, vasoconstriction an afterload increase. Therapeutic modulation of afterload is preformed via vasoactive pharmacological agents: vacoconstrictors increase afterload, vasodilators or ACE (Angiotensin Converting Enzyme) inhibitors, decrease afterload.

Similar to contractility, afterload is a systolic phenomenon; its timing coincides with the EPC.

4.2.2 Perfusion Blood Flow: Chronotropy Modulation

After **SI** is formed as a result of hemodynamic modulation by intravascular volume, inotropy and vasoactivity (see Fig.4.2.2), this blood flow/beat value is compared (by the brain) to a required tissue perfusion level performed by **CI** and, subsequently, by **DO₂I**. **HR** is the parameter, which ties these two conditions together. This activity is called the chronotropic compensation or chronotropic modulation.

This **chronotropic modulation** pathway by **HR** takes place at the Perfusion Blood Flow level (see Fig.4.2.2). In contrast to hemodynamic modulation, which is a **multivectorial** compensatory activity (each modulator exhibits both a magnitude and a direction), chronotropic modulation is a **scalar** (exhibits only a magnitude).

Definition of chronotropy, therefore, does not relate to an absolute level of HR but only how well this compensatory/modulating pathway accomplishes its task to achieve normal perfusion of all tissues.
Normochronotropy, therefore, is synonymous with a **normal value/range of CI**, **hypochronotropy** with an **infra-normal value of CI**, and **hyperchronotropy** with a **supra-normal value of CI**.

Documentation of a long-term function of chronotropic compensation to maintain adequate perfusion blood flow level is in Fig.4.2.6. In contrast to Fig.4.2.1, where the recordings of MAP, SI and HR represent instantaneous beat-by-beat values of these parameters over a short time period during which the subject was resting and his oxygen demand was constant, recordings of the same parameters in Fig.4.2.6 are the **sliding averages over a 200 heartbeat**

period (as to eliminate the beat-by-beat fluctuations visible in Fig.4.2.1).

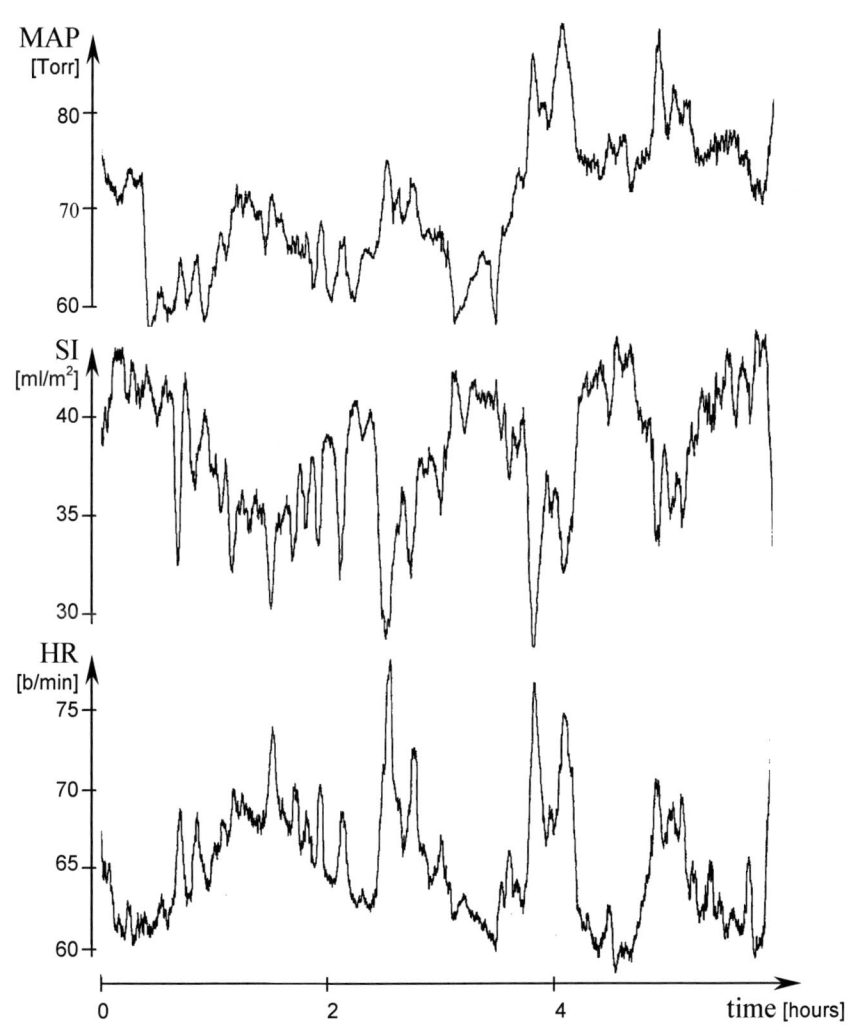

Fig.4.2.6: Sliding averages of MAP, SI and HR over a 6-hour period (courtesy of David Shannahoff-Khalsa, The Research Group for Mind-Body Dynamics, Institute for Nonlinear Science, University of California San Diego, California). The raw data were obtained in a beat-by-beat fashion during a sleep study and then subjected to the 200-beat sliding average calculation and plotting. These recordings document that in addition to the dynamic, beat-by-beat adjustments of HR to beat-by-beat variation of SI (as shown in Fig.4.2.1), the absolute value of HR continually adjusts to the absolute value of SI as well, in order to maintain CI at a level providing an adequate perfusion blood flow.

These recordings cover almost 6 hours during a sleep study during which the longer-term oxygen demand was not constant. The chronotropic modulation by HR, therefore, had to compensate both for the short-term fluctuations of SI (Mayer waves and respiration) and for the long-term variations of the absolute value of SI. Note that SI and HR are still close to being mirror images of each other, while, the MAP recording proves again that arterial blood pressure changes its value independently from SI due to an independent, beat-by-beat variation of vasoactivity.

4.2.3 Timing Considerations of Hemodynamic Modulation

Fig. 4.2.7 depicts the times of active phases of preload, contractility and afterload in respect to systolic and diastolic time intervals. See Fig.4.2.3 for timing definitions.

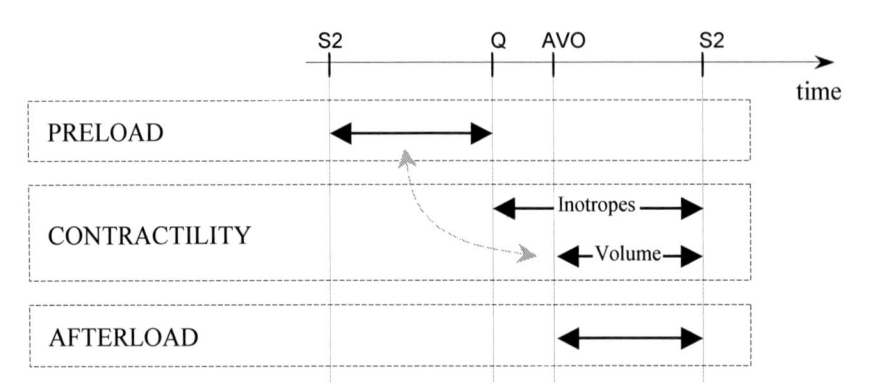

Fig.4.2.7: Timing considerations of working effects of **preload, contractility** (pharmacological = inotropes, and mechanical = Frank-Starling mechanism, i.e., effects of intravascular volume) and **afterload** in respect to Systolic and Diastolic Time Intervals: Diastole => Starts at S2-time, ends at Q-time. Systole => Isovolumic phase starts at Q-time, ends at AVO-time; Ejection phase starts at AVO-time, ends at S2-time.

5. Hemodynamic Management

5.1. Graphical Presentation of Hemodynamic State: The Hemodynamic Map

In geography, two coordinates - longitude and latitude - clearly define location of any point on earth. This well known graphical presentation is a geographic map.

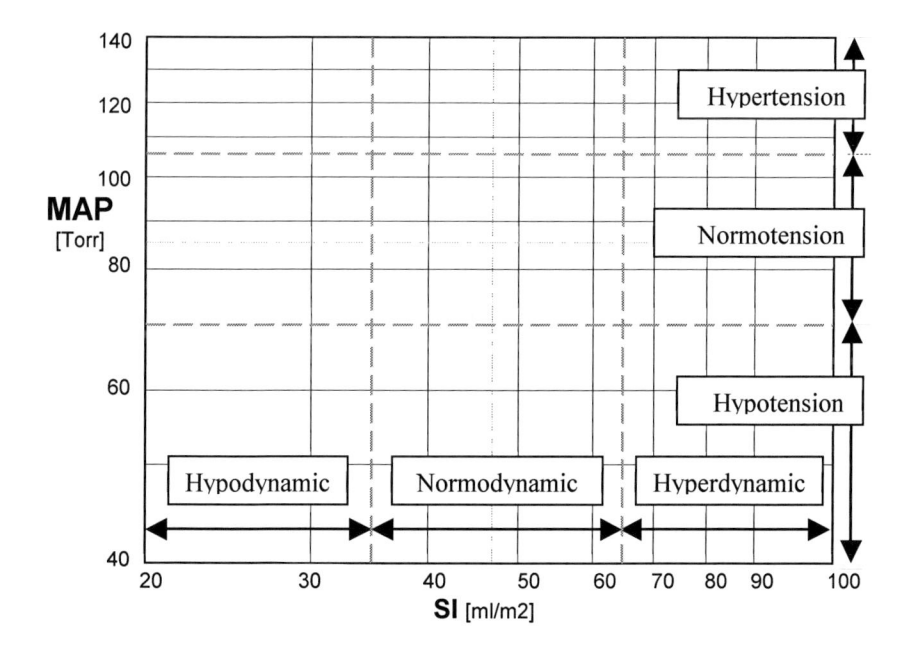

Fig.5.1: Hemodynamic map for supine, resting adults: SI is on the horizontal axis, MAP on the vertical one. A patient's hemodynamic point is located at the intersection of coordinates of **actual SI** and **MAP** values. Dot-and-dash lines mark the ideal hemodynamic values of SI = 47 ml/m^2 and MAP = 85 Torr. Two sets of dash lines mark normal ranges of SI (35 < SI < 65 ml/m^2) and MAP (70 < MAP < 105 Torr). Hypertensive, Normotensive and Hypotensive blood pressure bands, as well as Hypodynamic, Normodynamic and Hyperdynamic blood flow bands are marked, delineating a total of nine classes of hemodynamic states. Only one of them, a **simultaneous** Normodynamic and Normotensive state, called the **Normohemodynamic state**, is the desired hemodynamic state (Therapeutic Goal).

Since simultaneously measured SI and MAP define the hemodynamic state, a two-dimensional presentation of the hemodynamic state as a point on a **hemodynamic map** with coordinates of actual values of SI and MAP, is the easiest and most understandable description of a patient's hemodynamics.

Fig.5.1: SI is on the horizontal axis, MAP is on vertical. Normal ranges of SI are (35<SI<65 ml/m²)[3] and of MAP are (70<MAP< 105 Torr) [3]. They are marked by sets of dashed lines. Ideal values[3] of SI = 47 ml/m² and MAP = 85 Torr are marked by dot-and-dash lines. Please note that the hemodynamic map has a logarithmic scale. The reasons for logarithmic scale will be explained later in this Chapter.

A **patient's hemodynamic point**, defined by actual values of SI and MAP, can land within one of nine rectangles defining nine classes of hemodynamic states. Though three hemodynamic states are associated with normotension (hypodynamic normotensive, normodynamic normotensive and hyperdynamic normotensive states), only one of them - normodynamic normotensive state, called the **normohemodynamic state,** is the desired hemodynamic state, i.e., the **Therapeutic Goal.**

This presentation of hemodynamics also reveals the Achilles heel of the current flawed treatment of hypertension, which strives just for normotension and does not recognize that a hypodynamic normotensive patient and/or hyperdynamic normotensive patient are, actually, in abnormal hemodynamic states, which should be therapeutically treated.

As discussed in Chapter 4.2, the hemodynamic state is an end-result of multivectorial hemodynamic modulation by volume, inotropy and vasoactivity. From a physical viewpoint, the cardiovascular system acts as an interactive system that can be divided into two basic compartments interacting within each other:

(a) Compartment of the **pump;** its hemodynamic properties expressed as **contractility** and affected either by **intravascular volume** (preload) and/or by **inotropy.**
(b) Compartment of the **systemic vasculature;** its hemodynamic properties expressed as **afterload,** and affected by **vasoactivity.**

An explanation of vasoactivity (afterload) is a simpler task from the educational viewpoint. So we will start first with vasoactivity, which reflects the effects of the status of systemic vasculature back onto the pump and on systemic hemodynamics.

5.2 Hemodynamic Effects of Vasoactivity

Eq.4.4 defines the relationship between the vasoactive state (SSVRI value) and its modulating effect on a patient's hemodynamics, i.e., the SI and MAP values.

Ideal hemodynamic values for adults are[3]:

MAP_{ideal} = 85 Torr and SI_{ideal} = 47 ml/m^2 (the second order of magnitude hemodynamic parameter is the CVP_{ideal} = 4 Torr), resulting in an ideal value of $SSVRI_{ideal}$ = 137.8 dyn.sec.cm^{-5}.m^2.

The center of the hemodynamic map (the intersection of dot-and-dash lines of ideal values of MAP_{ideal} = 85 Torr and SI_{ideal} = 47 ml/m^2) in Fig.5.1, therefore, is also shared with the ideal value of vasoactivity ($SSVRI_{ideal}$ = 137.8 dyn.sec.cm^{-5}.m^2), although on a **different plane** than the plane of hemodynamic states. The isoline of SSVRI$_{ideal}$ = 137.8 dyn.sec.cm^{-5}.m^2, defined by an infinite number of SI and MAP pairs that produce this SSVRI value, is a straight line passing through the ideal normohemodynamic point from southwest to northeast; this line it is marked in Fig.5.2 as SSVRI = 137.8. Since this is an ideal SSVRI value, i.e., **ideal normovasoactivity**, its **deviation** from this ideal state **is marked** at its other end **as 0%**.

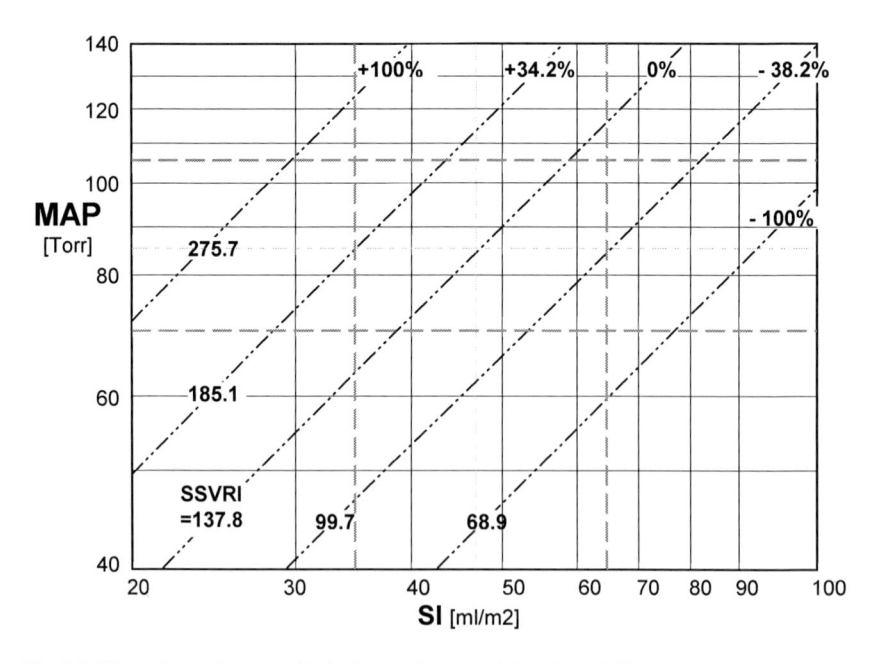

Fig.5.2: Hemodynamic map with isolines of vasoactivity plotted. The ideal normohemo-dynamic state of MAP$_{ideal}$ = 85 Torr and SI$_{ideal}$ = 47 ml/m^2 is also shared with the ideal value of vasoactivity SSVRI$_{ideal}$ = 137.8 dyn.sec.cm^{-5}.m^2, marked as 0% deviation in vasoactivity from ideal. Other isolines of vasoactivity plotted are: SSVRI = 185.1 (passing through ideal value of normotension MAP$_{ideal}$ = 85 and low end of normodynamic flow SI = 35), marked +34.2%, i.e., 34.2% vasoconstriction; SSVRI = 275.7 => +100%, i.e. 100% vasoconstriction; SSVRI = 99.7 => -38.2%, i.e., 38.2% vasodilation; and SSVRI = 68.0 => -100%, i.e., 100% vasodilation

Another isoline of vasoactivity plotted in Fig.5.2 is SSVRI = 185.1 dyn.sec. cm^{-5}.m^2. This isoline is passing through the ideal value of normotension MAP$_{ideal}$ = 85 and low end of range of normodynamic flow - SI = 35. When we compare this value of 185.1 to the ideal vasoactivity of 137.8 as 185.1/137.8 = 1.342, we can see that it is 34.2% **higher** than the ideal value, representing, therefore, a **34.2% vasoconstriction**. Similarly, an isoline of vasoactivity with a value of SSVRI = 275.7 represents 100% vasoconstriction (275.7/137.8 = 2).

When the values of calculated SSVRI are smaller than SSVRI$_{ideal}$ = 137.8 dyn.sec.cm^{-5}.m^2, the status of vasoactivity is **vasodilation**. For instance, SSVRI = 99.7, passing through the ideal value of normotension MAP$_{ideal}$ = 85 and high end of normodynamic blood flow SI = 65, represents a 38.2% vasodilation; and with a value of SSVRI = 68.0 represents a 100% vasodilation.

Similar to hemodynamic parameters, each having an ideal value and a band of normal values (for instance, ideal normotension is MAP$_{ideal}$ = 85 Torr, while the band of normotension is 70 < MAP < 105), even vasoactivity exhibits an ideal value (SSVRI$_{ideal}$) and a band of **normovasoactivity**. Normovasoactivity is formed by a band between isolines of SSVRI = 99.7 and SSVRI = 185.1 (i.e., 99.7<SSVRI< 185.1).

We can define normovasoactivity either mathematically as 99.7<SSVRI<185.1, or graphically, **when the hemodynamic point of a patient lands in a band between isolines of SSVRI = 99.7 and SSVRI = 185.1**.

EFFECTS OF **CVP** ON **SSVRI** CALCULATION:

If the CVP value is known (a patient is catheterized), its actual value is entered into the calculation of SSVRI (Eq.4.4). If noninvasive hemodynamic measurements are used and the actual value of CVP is unknown, the ideal value of CVP_{ideal} = 4 Torr is used in SSVRI calculations. Obviously, if the actual value of CVP differs from its ideal value of CVP_{ideal} = 4 Torr, there will be a difference (error) between the calculated and actual SSVRI value.

However, this error is minimal and negligible because:

- (a) When the normal value of CVP is compared to the normal value of MAP, we can see that CVP represents a parameter of the second order of magnitude (CVP << MAP), and,
- (b) when the patient is managed from an abnormal hemodynamic state into the normohemodynamic state and, as a result of hemodynamic management, SI and MAP approach their ideal values, we can assume that CVP will be approaching during this management process its ideal value as well. At the beginning of hemodynamic management, the only fact of importance is the **direction of therapy.** It does not make too much difference if the calculated deviation in vasoactivity is a 137% vasoconstriction and the actual status of vasoactivity (if CVP would be known) would be a 115% vasoconstriction. In either case the hemodynamic management direction for a clinician is clear – vasodilate!

In summary: Measuring a patient's SI and MAP values allows us to plot his hemodynamic point on the hemodynamic map. Position of this point in the sets of SSVRI coordinates (at a different plane), allows us to determine the deviation in vasoactivity from ideal, expressed either as normovasoactivity, or as a percentage deviation in vasoconstriction or as a percentage deviation in vasodilation.

5.3 Hemodynamic Effects of Intravascular Volume and Inotropy

We have already mentioned in Chapter 4.1 that in "per-minute" hemodynamics the contractility is not routinely assessed and its understanding is veiled in imprecise explanations.

As discussed previously, the hemodynamic modulating effects of both intravascular volume and inotropy affect the myocardial contractility (i.e., properties inherent to the pump), therefore, they must have the same hemodynamic **vectorial direction** (the hemodynamic vectors of the effects of volume and effects of inotropy are superimposed onto each other).

Let's review our knowledge and find out if we can reach simpler and more straightforward explanation and understanding of contractility.

The conclusions of Chapter 1 and Chapter 4.2.1.2 can be listed as follows:

- Values of hemodynamic parameters used in "per-beat" hemodynamics are their mean values over one heartbeat interval
- Contractility is a systolic phenomenon
- Contractility takes place during two systolic time phases: the isovolumic and the ejection phase
- Modulation by inotropy affects contractility during both isovolumic and ejection phase (during the entire mechanical systole)
- Inotropy can be measured by TEB as ISI and normal values of inotropy as a function of gender and age are known (Table 4.2)

- Modulation by intravascular volume affects the contractility of ejection phase only
- Myocardial O_2 is consumed only during the contraction phase (isovolumic + ejection phase)
- About 75% of myocardial O_2 is consumed during the isovolumic phase, the rest during the ejection phase.
- Myocardial O_2 consumption/heartbeat is represented by LSWI (Eq.4.5)

We can rephrase these statements the following way: Though the calculated value of LSWI is the mean value of left ventricular work over the entire heartbeat interval, the actual myocardial work expenditure takes place during the mechanical systole only. More contractile myocardium expends more physical work and, therefore, exhibits a higher value of LSWI and burns more oxygen. **LSWI thus parallels the mean value of myocardial contractility**. This proxy of myocardial contractility through LSWI, however, represents a sum of both contractilities, i.e., contractility of isovolumic phase and contractility of ejection phase. Since inotropy modulates contractility during the entire mechanical systole, and volume modulates through Frank-Starling mechanism only the contractility of ejection phase, LSWI represents the sum of contractility modulations **by intravascular volume and by inotropy**.

Inotropy can be measured today directly by TEB technology. This process is independent from hemodynamic acquisition of SI and MAP. We can, therefore, isolate the effects of intravascular volume from the effects of inotropy by solving two equations of two variables.

SSVRI and LSWI, representing two interactive compartments - systemic vasculature and the pump - are not only interesting dual interactive compartments from the physiologic viewpoint but represent dual parameters from a mathematical viewpoint as well: SSVRI, essentially, represents the **ratio** of MAP over SI, while the LSWI is their **prod-**

uct. Whereas **isolines of SSVRI** in hemodynamic map (Fig.5.2) **represent the status of vasoactivity, isolines of LSWI** (Fig.5.3) thus **describe the status of total myocardial contractility.**

Eq.4.5 defines the relationship between the myocardial contractile state (LSWI value) and its modulating effect on a patient's hemodynamics, i.e., the SI and MAP values. Ideal hemodynamic values for adults are[3]: MAP_{ideal} = 85 Torr and SI_{ideal} = 47 ml/m² (the second order of magnitude hemodynamic parameter is the $PAOP_{ideal}$ = 9 Torr), resulting in an ideal value of $LSWI_{ideal}$ = 52.8 g.m/m².

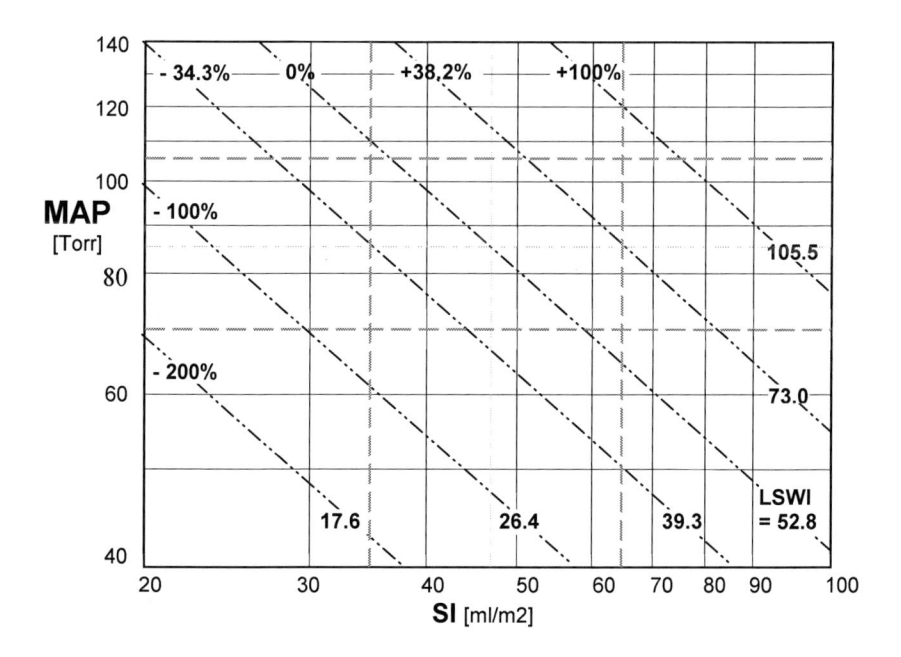

Fig.5.3: Hemodynamic map with isolines of contractility plotted. The ideal normohemodynamic state of MAP_{ideal} = 85 Torr and SI_{ideal} = 47 ml/m² is also shared with the ideal value of contractility $LSWI_{ideal}$ = 52.8 g.m/m², marked as 0% deviation in contractility from ideal. Other isolines of contractility plotted are: LSWI = 39.3 (passing through ideal value of normotension MAP_{ideal} = 85 and low end of normodynamic flow SI = 35), marked -34.3%, i.e., 34.3% hypocontractility; LSWI = 26.4 => -100%, i.e., 100% hypocontractility; LSWI = 73.0 => +38.2%, i.e., 38.2% hypercontractility; and LSWI = 105.5 => +100%, i.e., 100% hypercontractility

The center of the hemodynamic map (the intersection of dot-and-dash lines of ideal values of MAP_{ideal} = 85 Torr and SI_{ideal} = 47 ml/m^2) in Fig.5.3, therefore, is also shared with the ideal value of myocardial contractility ($LSWI_{ideal}$ = 52.8 g.m/m^2), although on a **different plane** than the plane of hemodynamic states. The isoline of $LSWI_{ideal}$ = 52.8 g.m/m^2, defined by an infinite number of SI and MAP pairs that produce this LSWI value, is, with a logarithmic scale of coordinates, a straight line (it would be a hyperbola if linear scale of coordinates would be used). This line is passing through the ideal normohemodynamic point from southeast to northwest; it is marked in Fig.5.3 as LSWI = 52.8. Since this is an ideal LSWI value, i.e., **ideal myocardial normocontractility**, its **deviation** from this ideal state **is marked** at its other end **as 0%**.

In summary: Measuring a patient's SI and MAP values allows us to plot his hemodynamic point on the hemodynamic map. Position of this hemodynamic point in the sets of LSWI coordinates (at a different plane), allows us to determine the deviation in contractility from ideal, expressed either as a percentage deviation in hypercontractility or as a percentage deviation in hypocontractility.

5.4 The Hemodynamic Management Chart

After reading the previous explanations, allowing us to express graphically the relationship between status of myocardial contractility and hemodynamic state and status of vasoactivity and hemodynamic state, you can surmise that these two modulating directions can be superimposed on each other. The result is the **Hemodynamic Management Chart for Adults** (Fig.5.4).

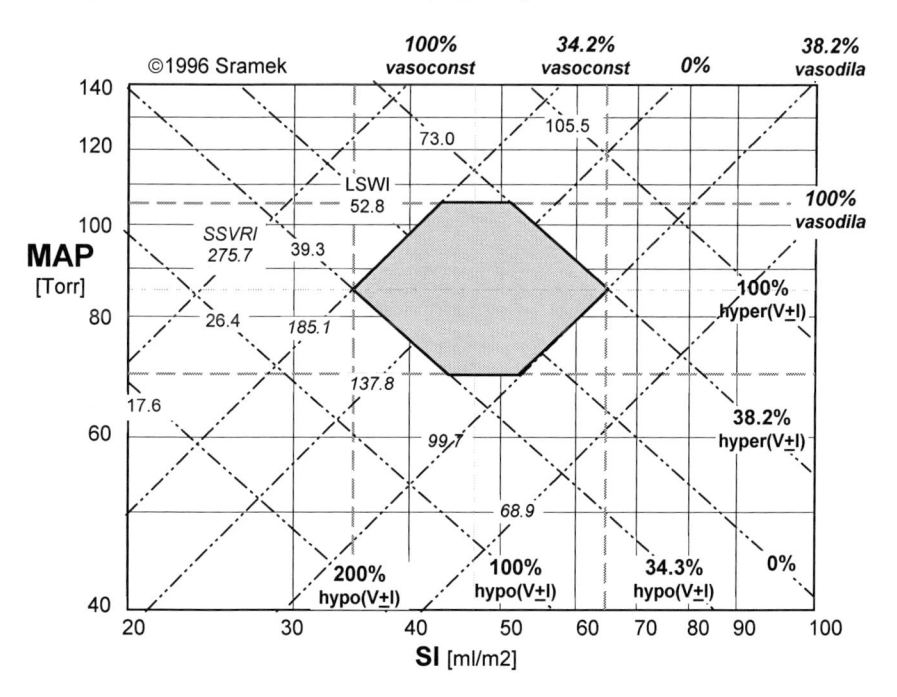

Fig.5.4: Hemodynamic Management Chart for supine, resting adults. Hemodynamic map is formed by the orthogonal system of coordinates. A map of hemodynamic modulators (an orthogonal system of coordinates on a different plane) is formed by sets of diagonal lines. Location of a patient's hemodynamic point is shared by both systems of coordinates. Its location within the map of hemodynamic modulators determines the status of hemodynamic modulators responsible for the hemodynamic state. The isolines of LSWI are the isolines of total myocardial contractility, representing the sum of modulating effect of volume and/or inotropy. Isolines of SSVRI (marked in Italic) are the isolines of vasoactivity. The loci of normohemodynamic states are defined by gray hexagon. Detailed explanation of the Chart is in text.

Superimposing Fig.5.1, Fig.5.2 and Fig.5.3 onto each other forms the **Hemodynamic Management Chart** for supine, resting adults. It consists of two maps, each having an orthogonal system of coordinates in its own plane. One is the Map of Hemodynamic Modulators (the causes); the other is the Hemodynamic Map (the consequence).

If the **Hemodynamic Map** is formed by the orthogonal system of coordinates (as in Fig.5.1), then the **Map of Hemodynamic Modulators** (an orthogonal system of coordinates on a different plane) is formed by sets of diagonal lines (as in Figs.5.2 and 5.3). These maps are interchangeable in their superimposed presentations, i.e., if the Map of Hemodynamic Modulators would be the orthogonal one, then the Hemodynamic Map would be formed by sets of diagonal lines.

Both maps share the location of a patient's hemodynamic point:

- Location of a patient's hemodynamic point within the Map of Hemodynamic Modulators determines the status of hemodynamic modulators responsible for the patient's hemodynamic state:

    The **isolines of LSWI are the isolines of total myocardial contractility, representing the vectorial sum of modulating effect of [volume ± Inotropy] (V±I).**

    Drawn in Fig.5.4 are the following **isolines of contractility:**

    (a) isolines delineating the band of normo(volemia ± inotropy) = normo(V±I), i.e., isoline 34.3% hypo(V±I), corresponding to LSWI = 39.3, and isoline 38.2% hyper(V±I), corresponding to LSWI = 73.0
    (b) 100% hyper(volemia ± inotropy) = hyper(V±I), corresponding to LSWI = 105.5

(c) 100% hypo(volemia ± inotropy) = hypo(V±I), corresponding to LSWI = 26.4, and
(d) 200% hypo(volemia ± inotropy) = hypo(V±I), corresponding to LSWI = 17.6

Note to Deviation in Volume and/or Inotropy:
We have already mentioned that the intravascular volume and inotropy are two modulators related to contractility, i.e., inherent property of the compartment of the pump. As such, they exhibit the same vectorial direction within the Hemodynamic Management Chart and are marked that way. Since the deviation in contractility represents their total vectorial sum, i.e. (V±I), we have to understand that, for example, a patient with his hemodynamic point located on the isoline of normocontractility (LSWI = 52.8) can be in this hemodynamic state either as a result of normovolemia and normoinotropy, however, also as a result of such a hemodynamic state, in which the deviation in volume and deviation in inotropy has each a finite deviation value but of an opposite sign, as for instance, a 43% hypovolemia accompanied with a 43% hyperinotropy. Similarly, a patient with 40% hypo(volemia ± inotropy) = 40% hypo(V±I), can be in this state while being normovolemic and 40% hypoinotropic.

Drawn in Fig.5.4 in the perpendicular direction are the following **isolines of vasoactivity** (marked in Fig.5.4 in Italic):

(a) isolines delineating the band of normovasoactivity, i.e., isoline of 38.2% vasodilation = 38.2% vasodila, corresponding to SSVRI = 99.7, and isoline of 34.2% vasoconstriction = 34.2% vasoconst, corresponding to SSVRI = 185.1,
(b) 100% vasodilation = 100% vasodila, corresponding to SSVRI = 68.9, and

(c) 100% vasoconstriction = 100% vasoconst, corresponding to SSVRI = 275.7

- Location of a patient's hemodynamic point within the Hemodynamic Map determines the patient's hemodynamic state.

   *The normohemodynamic state **is not** formed by the entire normotensive normodynamic rectangle in Fig.5.1, as one may expect, but by the gray hexagon inscribed within this rectangle, which contains loci of normohemodynamic states. In Fig.5.4, this hexagon is outlined by $MAP_{normal\text{-}max}$ and $MAP_{normal\text{-}min}$, and by isolines of contractility and vasoactivity passing through the MAP_{ideal} @ $SI_{normal\text{-}min}$ and MAP_{ideal} @ $SI_{normal\text{-}max}$.*

5.5 Hemodynamic Responses to Hemodynamic and Perfusion Blood Flow Management

The Hemodynamic Management Chart in Fig.5.4 does not only define the physiologic relationship between the statuses of hemodynamic modulators and hemodynamic state but allows us to understand and anticipate the hemodynamic responses to different hemodynamic manipulations:

- Volume expansion or volume reduction (diuresis) does not affect the status of vasoactivity. Therefore, these therapies will move the hemodynamic point along the corresponding isoline of vasoactivity the patient's hemodynamic point was residing on at the beginning of the therapy.

Volume expansion increases the SI value, while, at the same time, increasing the MAP value.
Volume reduction decreases the SI value, while, at the same time, decreasing the MAP value

- Positive or negative inotropic therapy does not affect the status of vasoactivity. Therefore, these therapies will move the hemodynamic point along the corresponding isoline of vasoactivity the patient's hemodynamic point was residing on at the beginning of the therapy.

Positive inotropes increase the SI value, while, at the same time, increasing the MAP value.
Negative inotropes decrease the SI value, while, at the same time, decreasing the MAP value.

- Vasoconstriction or vasodilation therapy does not affect the status of volume and/or inotropy. Therefore, these therapies will move the hemodynamic point along the corresponding isoline of volume and/or inotropy the patient's hemodynamic point was residing on at the beginning of the therapy.

Vasodilators increase the SI value, while, at the same time, decreasing the MAP value.
Vasoconstrictors decrease the SI value, while, at the same time, increasing the MAP value.

5.5.1 Calculations of Percentage Deviations in Intravascular Volume, Inotropy, Vasoactivity and Chronotropy from their Respective Ideal States

In all calculations of deviations, a **band** of certain percentage deviations straddling the ideal value of hemodynamic or perfusion flow modulator is considered to be the modulator's **normal range**.

5.5.1.1 Calculation of Percentage Deviation in Inotropy (ΔIno)

Ideal values of the TEB measurement of inotropic state (ISI_{ideal}) for supine, resting adults as a function of gender and age are listed in Table 4.2.

If **ISI** > **ISI**$_{ideal}$, the following equation for calculation of percentage deviation in inotropy (+ΔIno) is used and the calculated deviation is listed as "% **hyperinotropy**":

$$+\Delta Ino = [(ISI/ISI_{ideal}) - 1] \times 100\%$$

If **ISI** < **ISI**$_{ideal}$, the following equation for calculation of percentage deviation in inotropy (-ΔIno) is used and the calculated deviation is listed as "% **hypoinotropy**":

$$-\Delta Ino = [(ISI_{ideal}/ISI) - 1] \times 100\%$$

If **0.833 ISI**$_{ideal}$ < **ISI** < **1.2 ISI**$_{ideal}$, then the inotropic status is listed as "**normoinotropy**."

5.5.1.2 Calculation of Percentage Deviation in Intravascular Volume (ΔVol)

Solving two equations of two variables allows the determination of **Percentage Deviation in Intravascular Volume (ΔVol)** from ideal normovolemia:

(1) Determination of Percentage Deviation in Myocardial Contractility (ΔCon) from ideal (ideal value of LSWI for supine, resting adults is listed in Eq.4.5):

If **LSWI > LSWI** ideal, the following equation for calculation of percentage deviation in contractility (+ΔCon) is used:

$$+\Delta Con = [(LSWI / LSWI_{ideal}) - 1] \times 100\%$$

If LSWI < LSWI ideal, the following equation for calculation of percentage deviation in contractility (-ΔCon) is used:

$$-\Delta Con = -[(LSWI_{ideal} / LSWI) - 1] \times 100\%$$

(2) Determination of Percentage Deviation in Intravascular Volume (ΔVol) from ideal normovolemia:

When both **ΔCon** and **ΔIno** are known, then the Percentage Deviation in Intravascular Volume from ideal normovolemia is calculated as (the signs of ΔCon and ΔIno <u>must</u> be honored):

$$\Delta Vol = (\Delta Con) - (\Delta Ino)$$

If ΔVol is within a band of ± 20% of ΔVol_ideal, then the percentage deviation in volume is listed as **"normovolemia."**

If ΔVol ≥ +21%, then the percentage deviation in volume is listed as **"% hypervolemia."**

If ΔVol ≤ 21%, then the percentage deviation in volume is listed as **"% hypovolemia."**

Examples:

- *ΔC = +83%, ΔIno = +17%,
  then ΔVol = 66% hypervolemia*

- *ΔC = -33%, ΔIno = -17%,
  then ΔVol = normovolemia*

- *ΔC = +23%, ΔIno = +17%,
  then ΔVol = normovolemia*

- *ΔC = -23%, ΔIno = +17%,
  then ΔVol = 40% hypovolemia*

- *ΔC = -83%, ΔIno = -17%,
  then ΔVol = 66% hypovolemia*

5.5.1.3 Calculation of Percentage Deviation in Vasoactivity (ΔVas)

Ideal values of the measure of vasoactivity, i.e., SSVRI_ideal, for supine, resting adults are listed in Eq.4.4.

If **SSVRI > SSVRI_ideal**, the following equation for calculation of percentage deviation in vasoactivity (+ΔVas) is used and the calculated deviation is listed as "% **vasoconstriction**":

$$+\Delta Vas = [(SSVRI/SSVRI_{ideal}) - 1] \times 100\%$$

If **SSVRI < SSVRI**$_{ideal}$, the following equation for calculation of percentage deviation in vasoactivity (-ΔVas) is used and the calculated deviation is listed as "% **vasodilation**":

$$-\Delta Vas = [(SSVRI_{ideal}/SSVRI) - 1] \times 100\%$$

If **0.833 SSVRI**$_{ideal}$ **< SSVRI < 1.2 SSVRI**$_{ideal}$, then the inotropic status is listed as "**normovasoactivity**"

5.5.1.4 Calculation of Percentage Deviation in Chronotropy (ΔChr)

As it was already discussed in Chapter 4.2.2, the definition of chronotropy does not relate to an absolute level of HR but only how well is this compensatory/modulating pathway accomplishing its task to achieve normal perfusion blood flow level, i.e., normal value of CI.

Ideal values of CI are listed in Chapter 2: For supine, resting adults is CI_{ideal} = 3.5 l/min/m². For surgical patients in the postoperative period (1-36 hours) after a major surgery, CI_{ideal} = 4.5 l/min/m².

If **CI > CI**$_{ideal}$, the following equation for calculation of percentage deviation in chronotropy (+ΔChr) is used and the calculated deviation is listed as "% **hyperchronotropy**":

$$+\Delta Chr = [(CI/CI_{ideal}) - 1] \times 100\%$$

If **CI < CI**ideal, the following equation for calculation of percentage deviation in chronotropy (-ΔChr) is used and the calculated deviation is listed as "% **hypochronotropy**":

$$-\Delta Chr = [(CI_{ideal}/CI) - 1] \times 100\%$$

If **0.833 CI**ideal **< CI < 1.2 CI**ideal, then the chronotropic status is listed as "**normochronotropy.**"

6. Normal Hemodynamic, O_2 Delivery and TEB Values in Neonatal and Pediatric Patients

This Chapter is, essentially, a transcript of scientific paper of the same title[23] by B. Bo Sramek, International Hemodynamic Society, and Viktor Hraska, Pediatric Cardiocentrum, Bratislava, Slovakia, presented at the 4th International Conference on Hemodynamics of the International Hemodynamic Society, 1998, Acapulco, Mexico.

Current hemodynamic data acquisition tools for neonatal and pediatric (N/P) patients are limited to monitoring ECG, pulse oximetry (SpO_2) and noninvasive blood pressure (NIBP).

With the exception of research facilities, the catheterization and resulting determination of cardiac output and oxygen delivery dynamics (DO_2I) in this special subgroup of patients is almost nonexistent.

Though normal values of all hemodynamic parameters and their normal ranges exist for adults[3], the information on normal values of hemodynamic parameters in neonates and pediatric patients as a function of age is scarce.

The following plots of normal neonatal and pediatric data include normal body habitus data and normal values of hemodynamic, oxygen delivery and TEB parameters. They are presented as a function of age from birth to 15 years of age:

- **Parameters compiled from neonatal/pediatric literature** are plotted in Figs.6.1, 6.2, 6.4, 6.6, 6.7, 6.8 and 6.9.

- **Parameters measured** on a large group of neonatal and pediatric patients with the TEB technology are plotted in Figs.6.10 and 6.13.

- **Parameters calculated** are:
  Fig.6.3 (Eq.2.2a), Fig.6.5 (Eq.2.4 & Figs.6.4 and 6.6 @ $SaO_2 \geq 95\%$), Fig.6.11 (Eq.4.5 & Figs.6.8 and 6.9 @ LAP = 7 Torr) and Fig.6.12 (Eq.4.4 & Figs.6.8 and 6.9 @ CVP = 4).

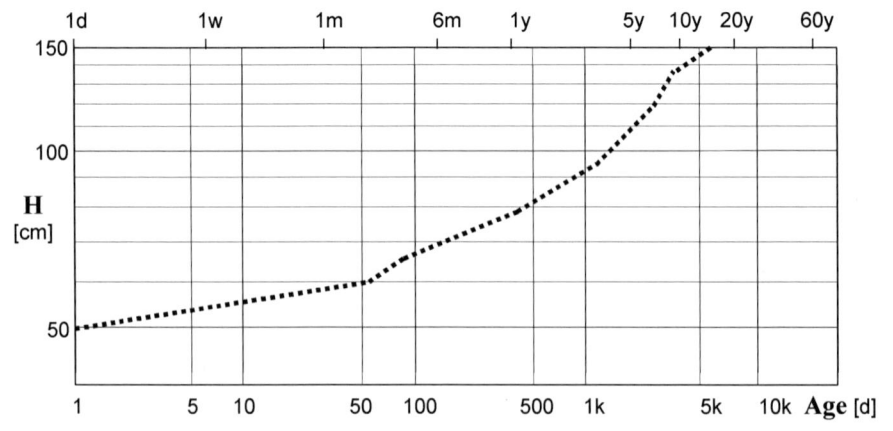

Fig.6.1: Normal **Height (H)** [cm] as a function of age in neonatal/pediatric patients. Bottom time scale has age in days (d), the top time scale in days (d), weeks (w), months (m) and years (y)

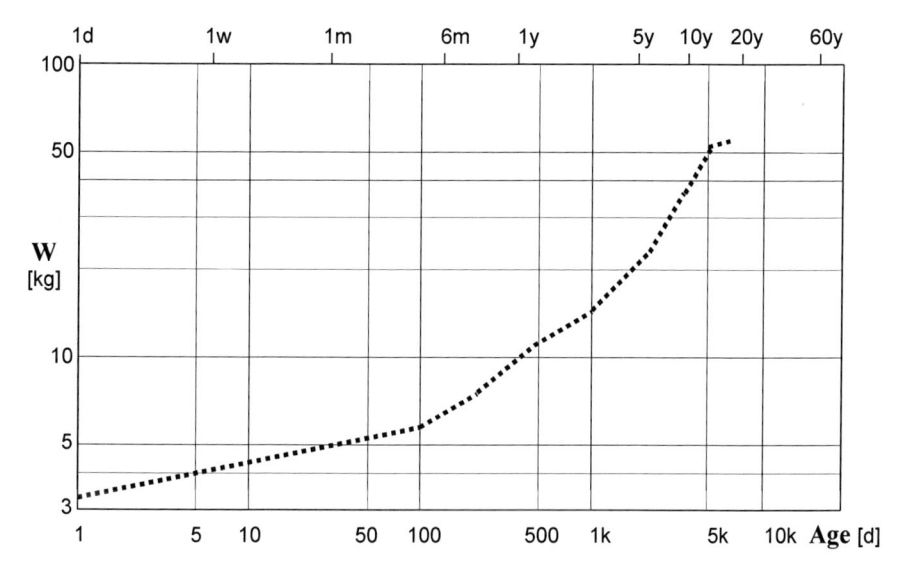

Fig.6.2: Normal **Weight (W)** [kg] as a function of age in neonatal/pediatric patients. Bottom time scale has age in days (d), the top time scale in days (d), weeks (w), months (m) and years (y)

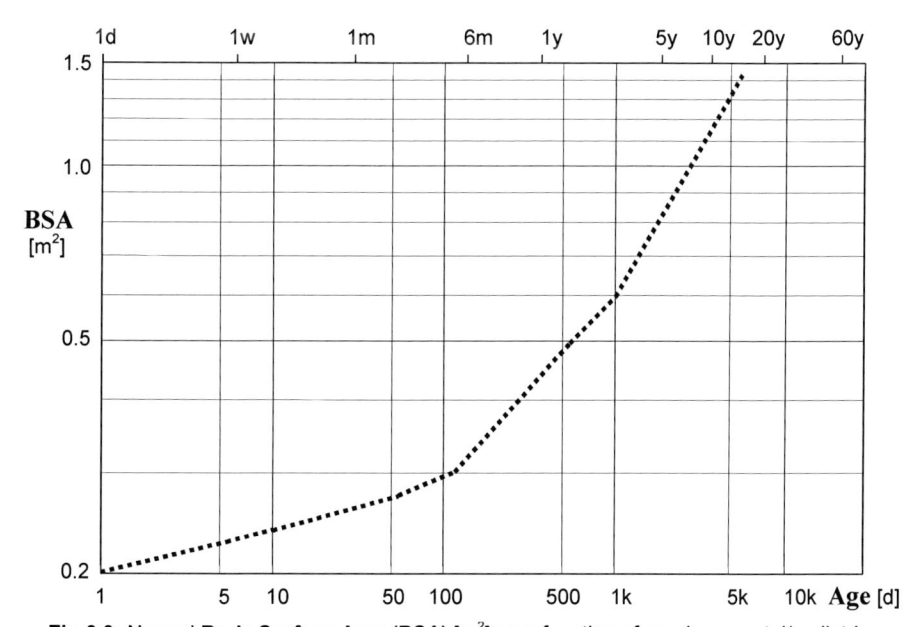

Fig.6.3: Normal **Body Surface Ares (BSA)** [m^2] as a function of age in neonatal/pediatric patients. Bottom time scale has age in days (d), the top time scale in days (d), weeks (w), months (m) and years (y)

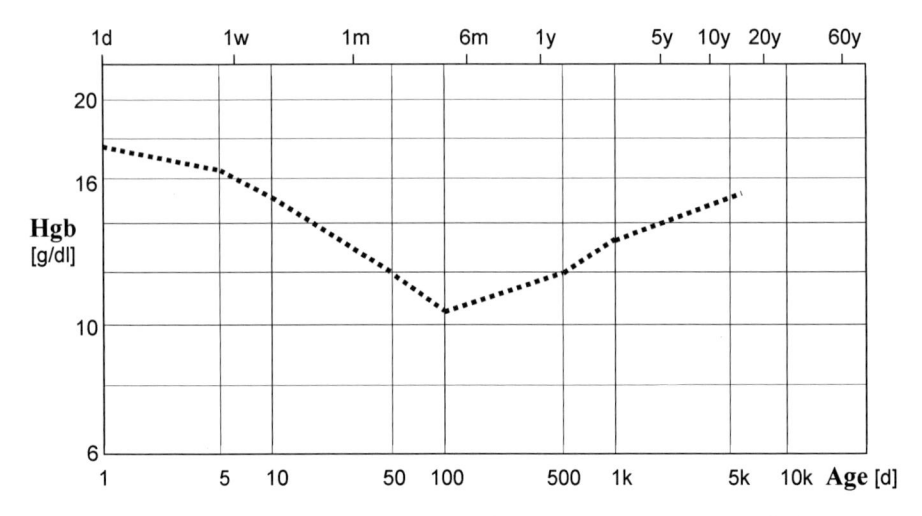

Fig.6.4: Normal **Hemoglobin (Hgb)** [g/dl] as a function of age in neonatal/pediatric patients. Bottom time scale has age in days (d), the top time scale in days (d), weeks (w), months (m) and years (y)

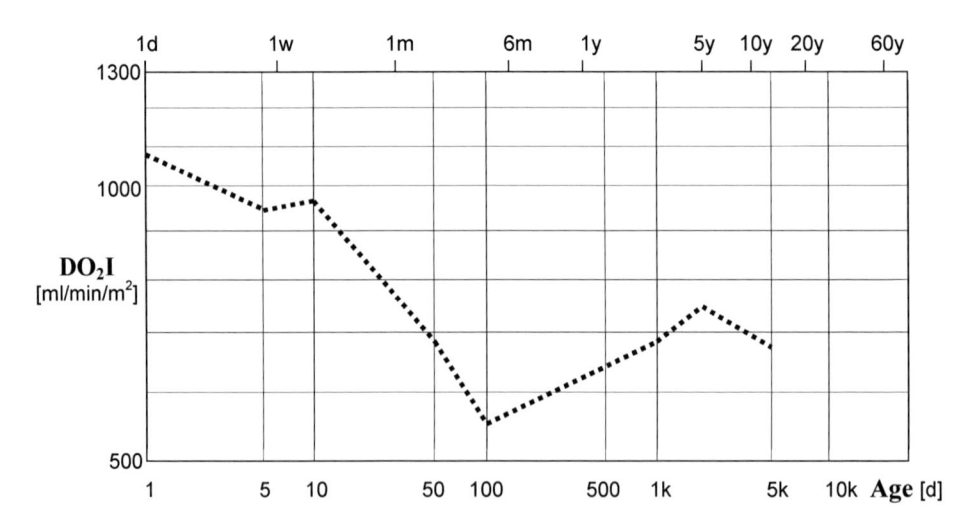

Fig.6.5: Normal **Oxygen Delivery Index (DO$_2$I)** [ml/min/m^2] as a function of age in neonatal/pediatric patients. Bottom time scale has age in days (d), the top time scale in days (d), weeks (w), months (m) and years (y)

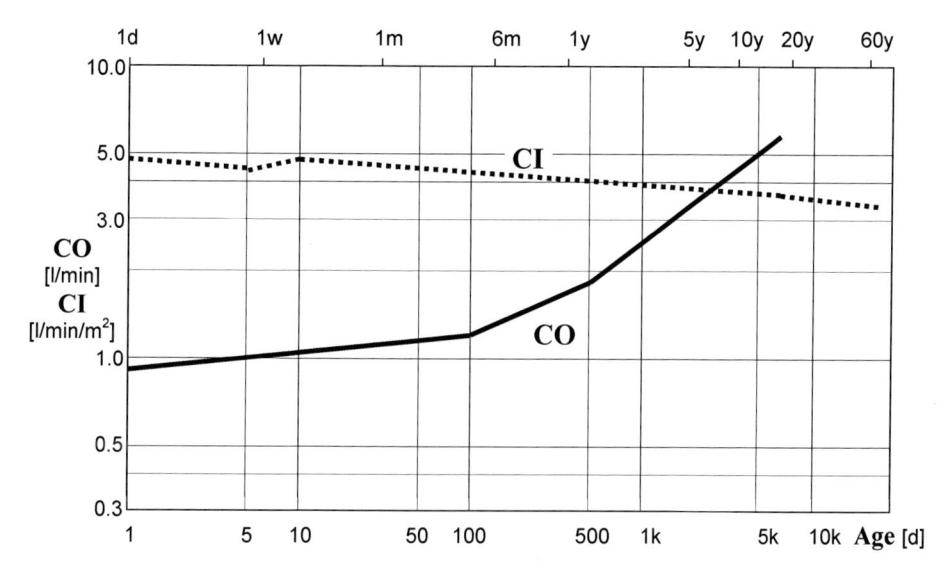

Fig.6.6: Normal **Cardiac Output (CO)** [l/min] and **Cardiac Index (CI)** [l/min/m^2] as a function of age in neonatal/pediatric patients. Bottom time scale has age in days (d), the top time scale in days (d), weeks (w), months (m) and years (y)

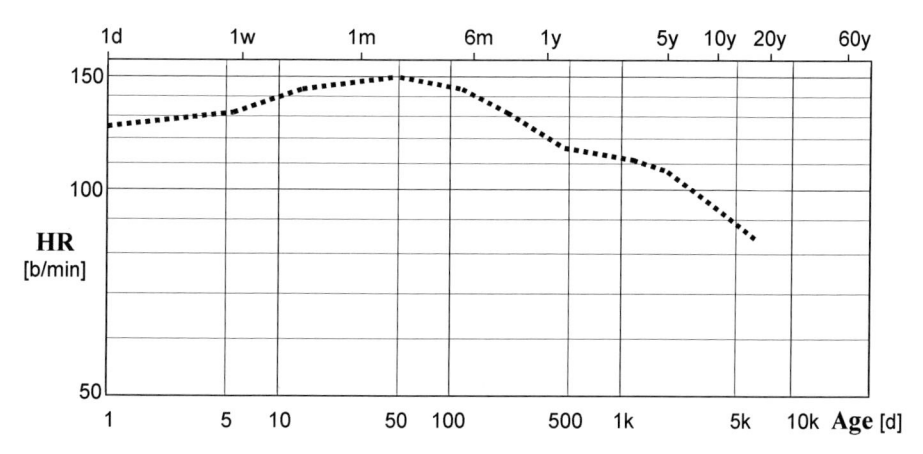

Fig.6.7: Normal **Hart Rate (HR)** [beats/min] as a function of age in neonatal/pediatric patients. Bottom time scale has age in days (d), the top time scale in days (d), weeks (w), months (m) and years (y)

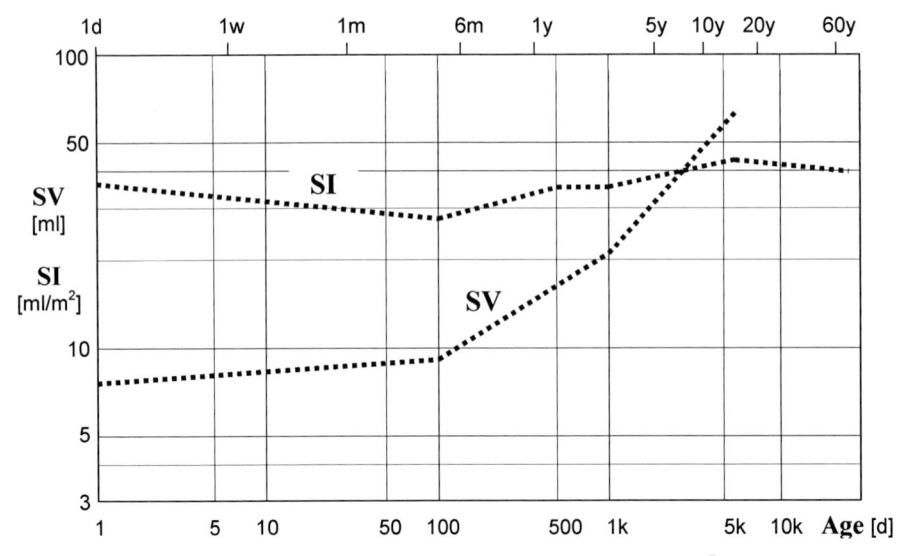

Fig.6.8: Normal **Stroke Volume (SV)** [ml] and **Stroke Index (SI)** [ml/m^2] as a function of age in neonatal/pediatric patients. Bottom time scale has age in days (d), the top time scale in days (d), weeks (w), months (m) and years (y)

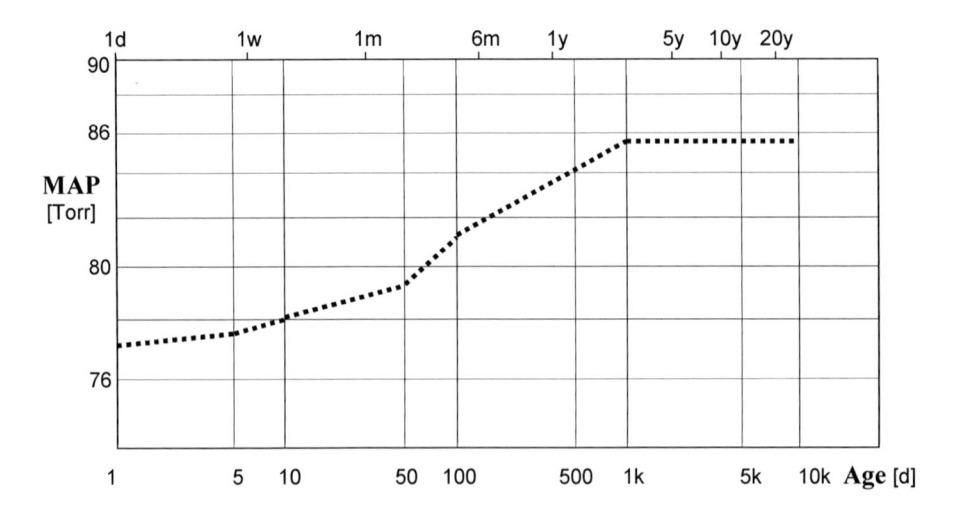

Fig.6.9: Normal **Mean Arterial Pressure (MAP)** [Torr = mmHg] as a function of age in neonatal/pediatric patients. Bottom time scale has age in days (d), the top time scale in days (d), weeks (w), months (m) and years (y)

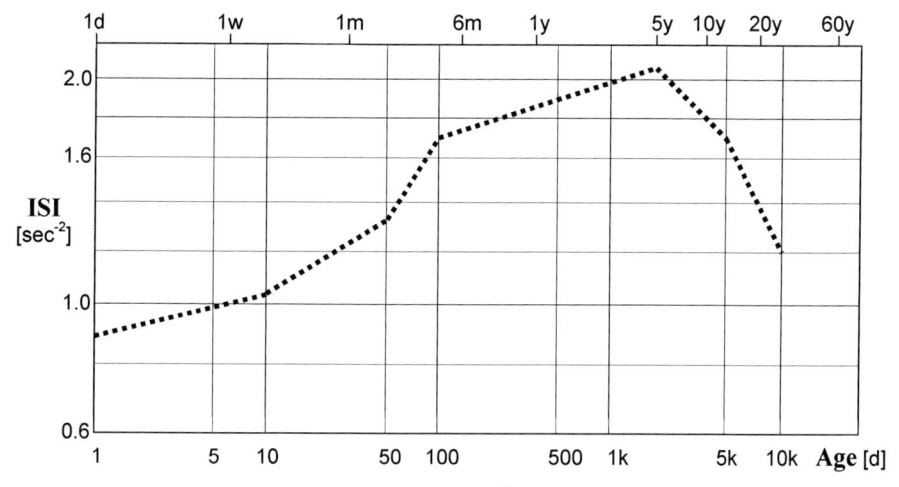

Fig.6.10: Normal **Inotropic State Index (ISI)** [sec^{-2}] as a function of age in neonatal/pediatric patients. Bottom time scale has age in days (d), the top time scale in days (d), weeks (w), months (m) and years (y)

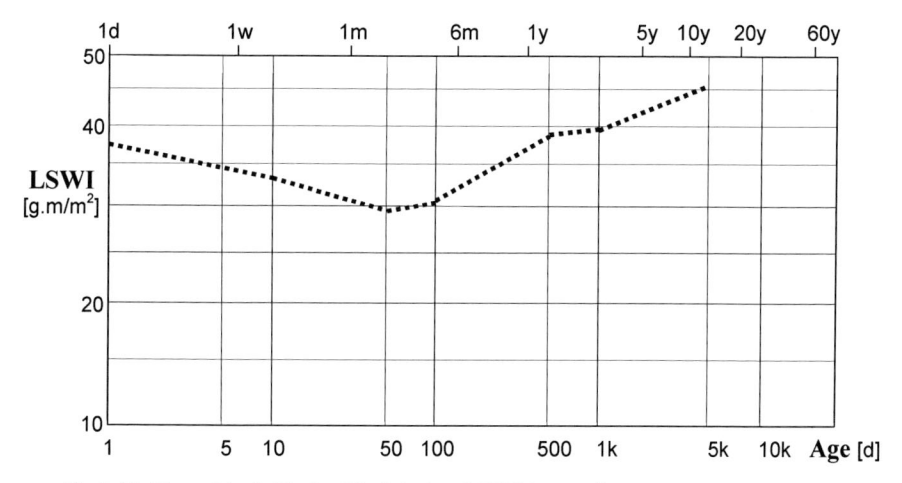

Fig.6.11: Normal **Left Stroke Work Index (LSWI)** [$g.m/m^2$] as a function of age in neonatal/pediatric patients. Bottom time scale has age in days (d), the top time scale in days (d), weeks (w), months (m) and years (y)

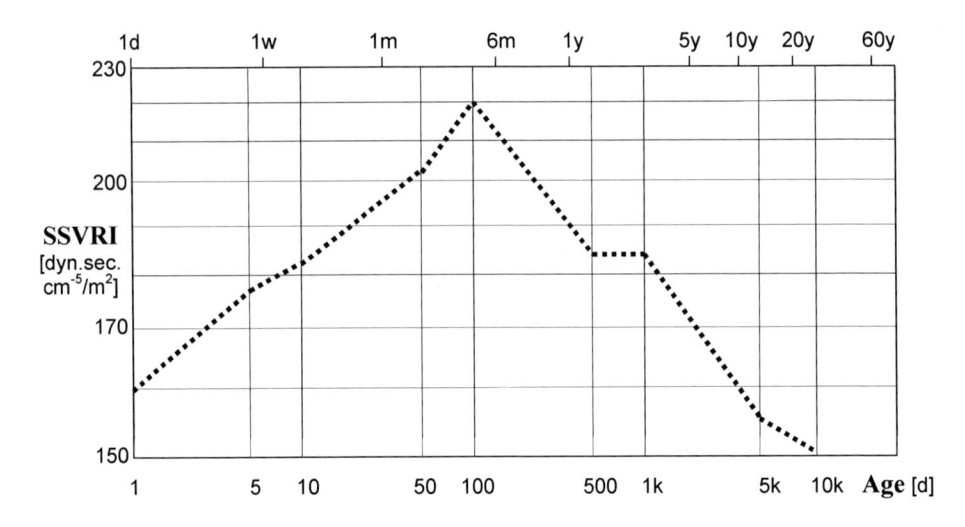

Fig.6.12: Normal **Stroke Systemic Vascular Resistance Index (SSVRI)** [dyn.sec.cm^{-5}/m^2] as a function of age in neonatal/pediatric patients. Bottom time scale has age in days (d), the top time scale in days (d), weeks (w), months (m) and years (y)

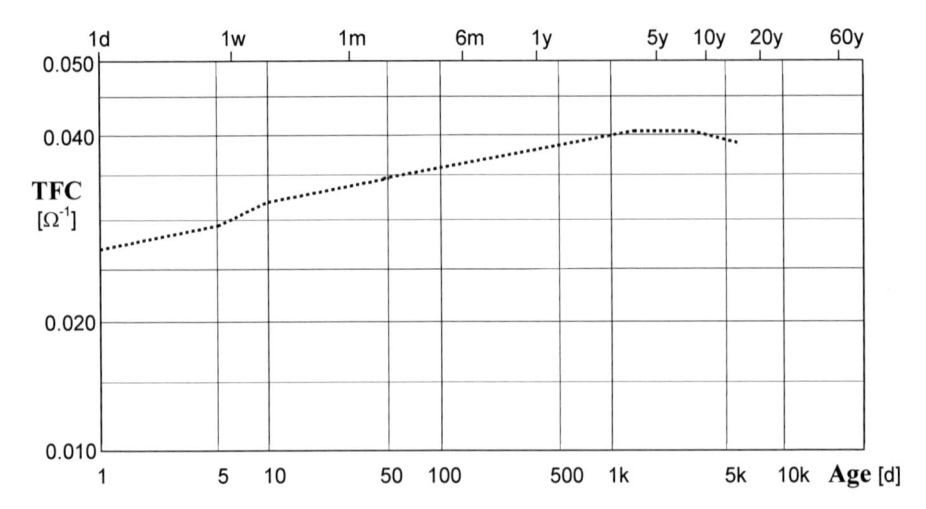

Fig.6.13: Normal **Thoracic Fluids Conductivity (TFC)** [1/Ω] as a function of age in neonatal/pediatric patients. Bottom time scale has age in days (d), the top time scale in days (d), weeks (w), months (m) and years (y)

Though the above-presented normal values of hemodynamic, perfusion blood flow and oxygen delivery parameters are for supine and resting neonates and pediatric patients, we can safely stipulate, that these patients, if undergoing a major surgery, should, similarly to their adult counterparts discussed in Chapter 2, be managed in the immediate postoperative period (1-36 hours) into the **Postoperative Therapeutic Goal**. The parameters affected by the immediate postoperative state are CI, DO_2I and VO_2I, which should be during this period about 30% higher than their corresponding normal values published in this chapter.

7. Normal Hemodynamic, O_2 Delivery and TEB Values in Gravidas and Nongravidas

This Chapter is a transcript of a paper of the same title[24] by B. Bo Sramek of the International Hemodynamic Society, and Kamila Nouzova and Antonin Parizek of Foundation Vita et Futura, Prague, Czech Republic, presented at the 4th International Conference on Hemodynamics of the International Hemodynamic Society, Acapulco, Mexico, 1998.

Current routine hemodynamic assessment tools for gravidas and nongravidas are limited to monitoring ECG, noninvasive blood pressure (NIBP) and, sometimes, pulse oximetry (SpO_2). The catheterization and resulting determination of CI and oxygen delivery dynamics (DO_2I) in this special subgroup of patients is almost nonexistent. As a result, many hemodynamic abnormalities are detected only when they reach their catastrophic stage. However, the noninvasive nature of Thoracic Electrical Bioimpedance (TEB) technology, in conjunction with NIBP and SpO_2 technologies, now allow us to measure complete hemodynamics and oxygen delivery dynamics in all women of childbearing age and during pregnancy.

To hemodynamically assess and manage the gravidas and nongravidas, we have to know normal values of other parameters as a function of gestation time (for nongravidas, the gestation time = 0), have to measure their complete hemodynamics (MAP & SI), perfusion blood flow dynamics (CI) and oxygen delivery dynamics (DO_2I), and determine normal values of hemodynamic modulators. By implementing novel concepts of hemodynamic management, we then can continually maintain these patients in normohemodynamic and normoperfusion state.

Following normal values of hemodynamic and O_2 delivery parameters, collected on a large group of gravidas and nongravidas with NIBP and TEB technologies, are presented as a function gestation time. Generally, normal ranges of all hemodynamic and oxygen delivery parameters form a band of ±20% from their respective ideal values presented in the graph.

- **Normal value of Hgb** during pregnancy was obtained from literature and is plotted in Fig. 7.2.
- **Parameters measured** on a large group of gravidas and nongravidas with the TEB and NIBP technologies are plotted in Figs.7.3-7.7.
- **Parameters calculated** are:
  Fig.7.1 (Eq.2.4 & Figs.7.2 and 7.3 @ $SaO_2 \geq 95\%$), Fig.7.8 (Eq.4.5 & Figs.7.6 and 7.7 @ LAP = 7 Torr) and Fig.7.9 (Eq.4.4 & Figs.7.6 and 7.7 @ CVP = 4).

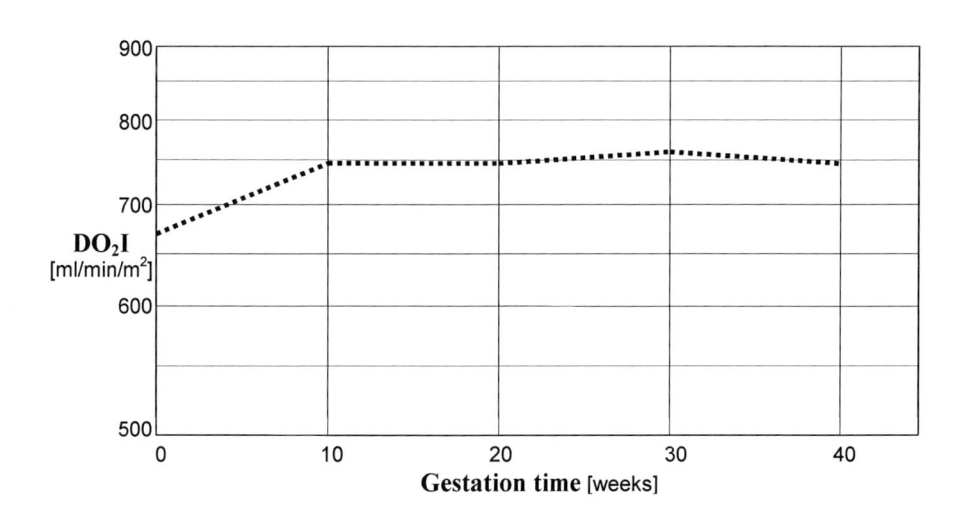

Fig.7.1: Normal value of **Oxygen Delivery Index (DO2I)** [ml/min/m^2] as a function of gestation time. For nongravidas, the gestation time = 0.

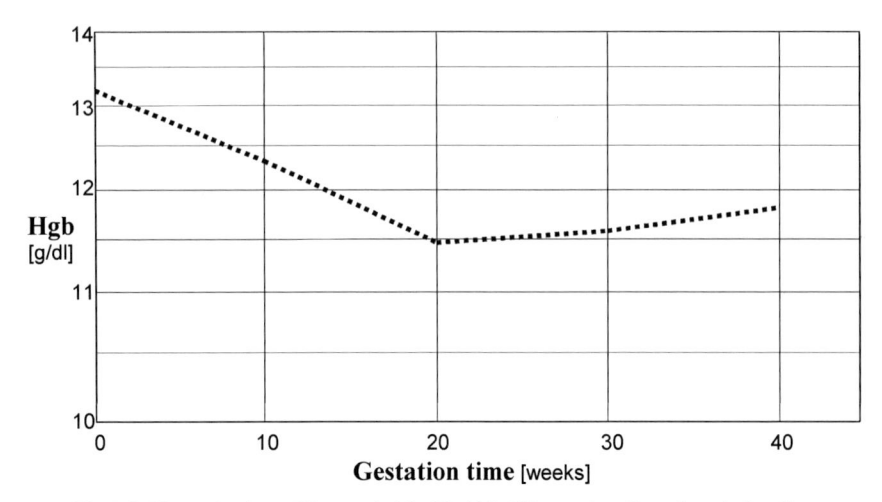

Fig.7.2: Normal value of **Hemoglobin (Hgb)** [g/dl] as a function of gestation time. For nongravidas, the gestation time = 0.

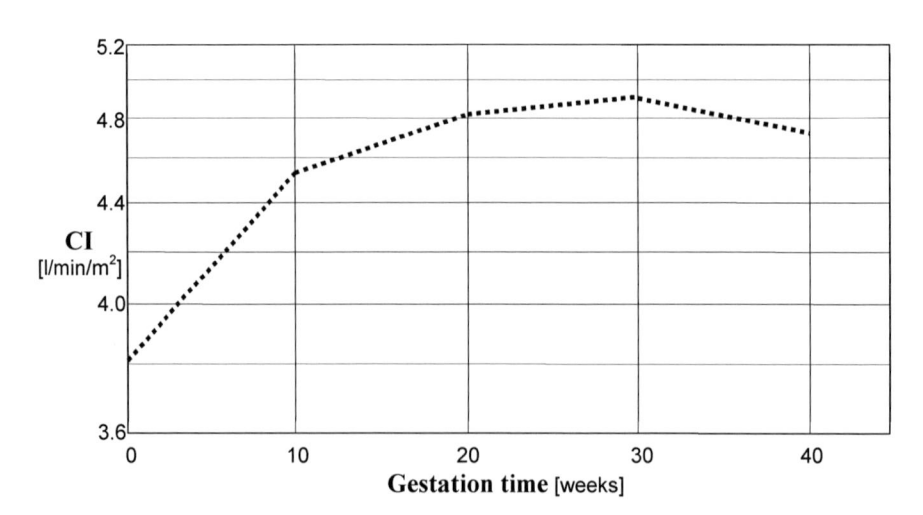

Fig.7.3: Normal value of **Cardiac Index (CI)** [l/min/m^2] as a function of gestation time. For nongravidas, the gestation time = 0.

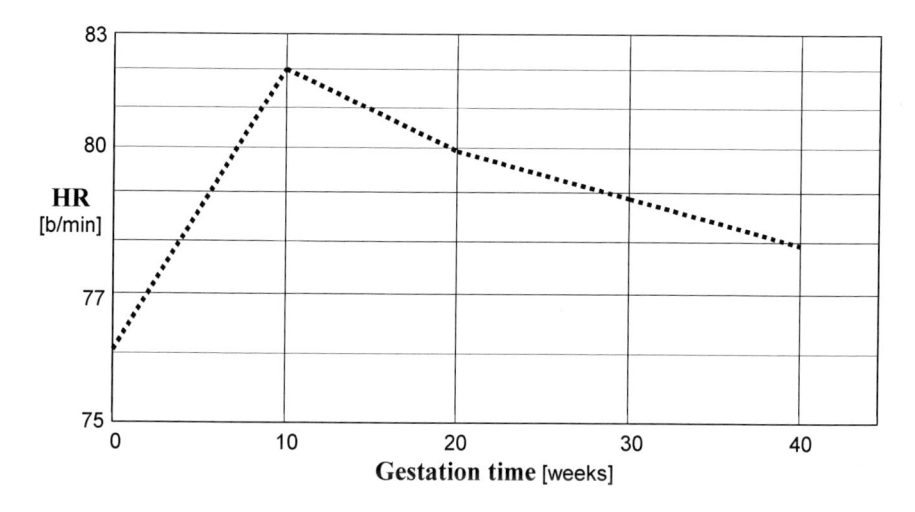

Fig.7.4: Normal value of **Heart Rate (HR)** [b/min] as a function of gestation time. For nongravidas, the gestation time = 0.

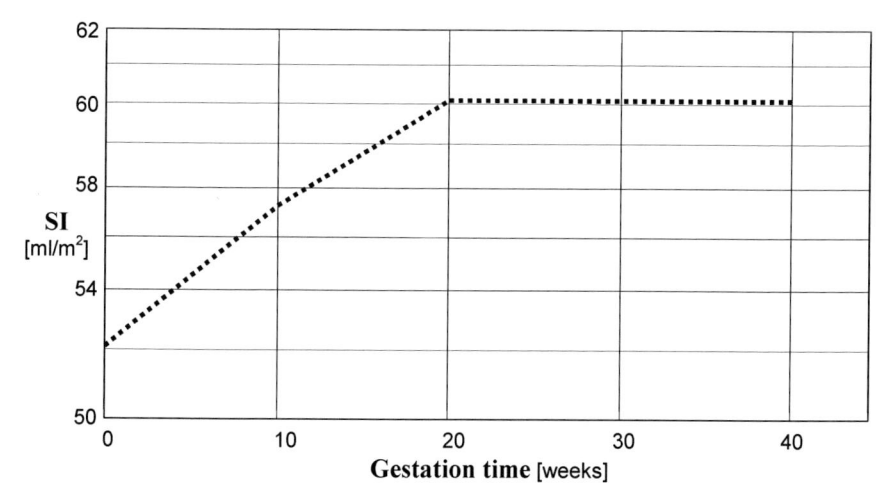

Fig.7.5: Normal value of **Stroke Index (SI)** [ml/m^2] as a function of gestation time. For nongravidas, the gestation time = 0.

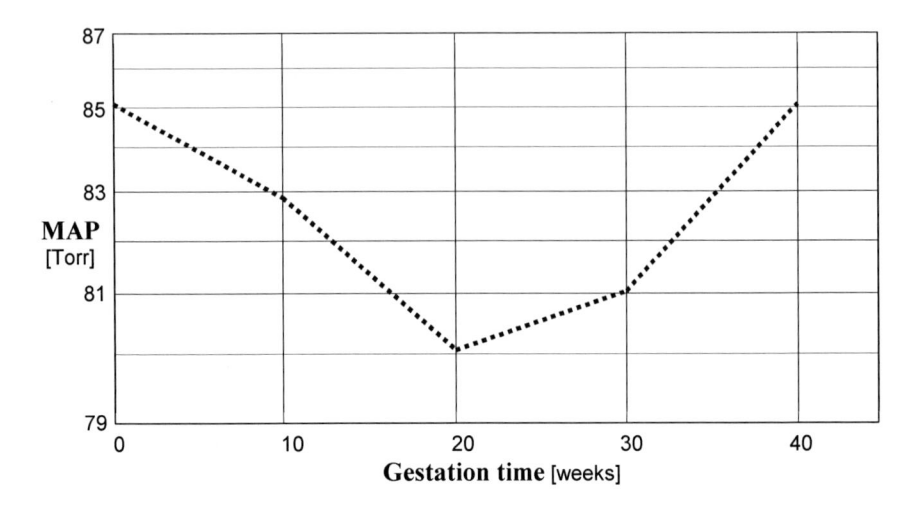

Fig.7.6: Normal value of **Mean Arterial Pressure (MAP)** [Torr] as a function of gestation time. For nongravidas, the gestation time = 0.

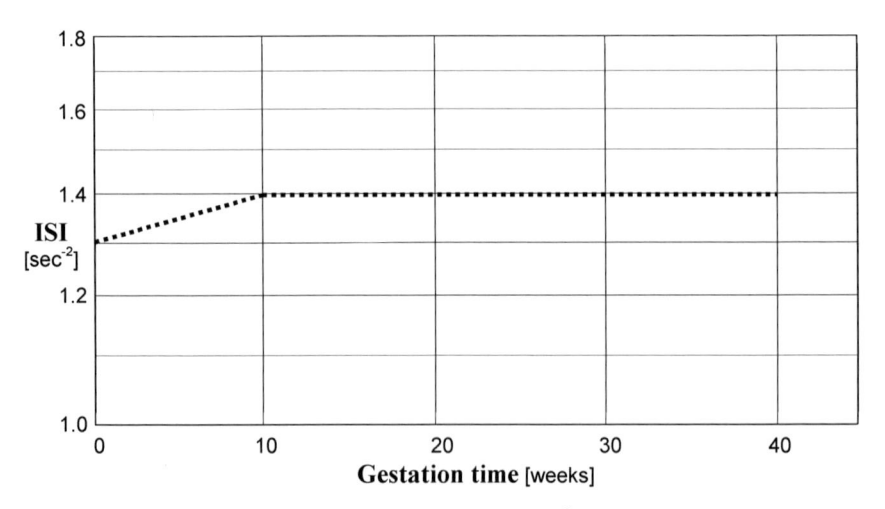

Fig.7.7: Normal value of **Inotropic State Index (ISI)** [sec^{-2}] as a function of gestation time. For nongravidas, the gestation time = 0.

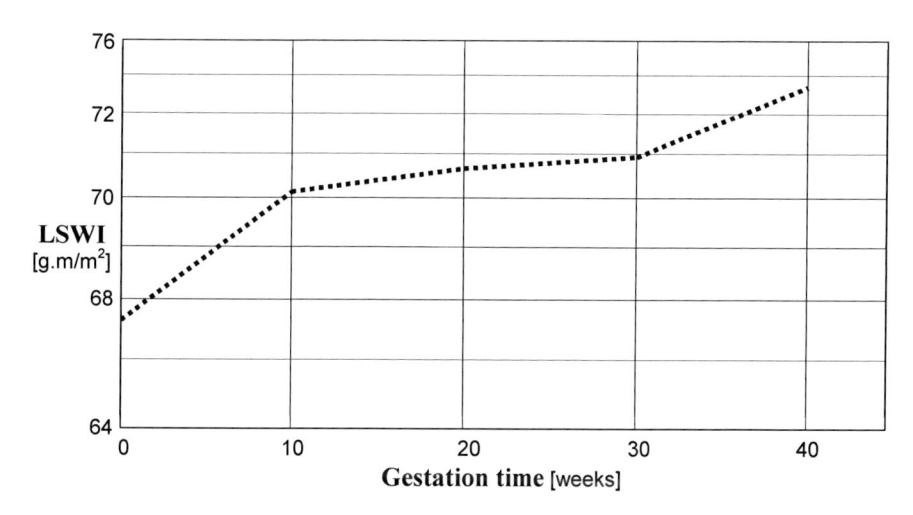

Fig.7.8: Normal value of **Left Stroke Work Index (LSWI)** [g.m/m^2] as a function of gestation time. For nongravidas, the gestation time = 0.

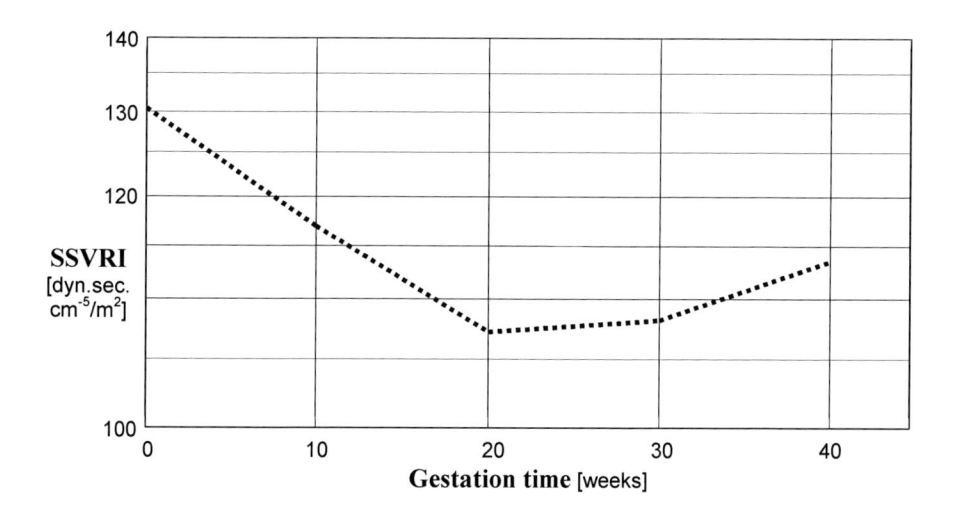

Fig.7.9: Normal value of **Stroke Systemic Vascular Resistance Index (SSVRI)** [dyn.sec.cm^{-5}/m^2] as a function of gestation time. For nongravidas, the gestation time = 0.

8. Hemodynamic Management with "Per-beat" Hemodynamics: Case Studies

8.1. Hemodynamic Management of a Surgical Patient in the ICU

Data for this case study have been provided courtesy of HEMO SAPIENS® INC (www.hemosapiens.com; visit this web site if you want to see examples of the following screen images used in this chapter in color). Its HOTMAN™ F111 System, used in this study, has the per-beat hemodynamics and hemodynamic management method, described in Chapter 5, implemented in its software.

This 24-minute case study documents the hemodynamic and oxygen transport management capability of per-beat hemodynamics methodology in the **intensive care setting.**

The patient was a 69-year old female who underwent a mitral valve replacement surgery. She was transported from the operating room into the intensive care unit at about 10:00 on October 31, 1996. The patient was managed by conventional means based upon information obtained from the patient monitor (HR, MAP & S/D blood pressures) and from the thermodilution (TD) catheter. The TD catheter was used to measure the values of CI, CVP and PAOP, and to periodically draw a sample of the mixed venous blood. The SvO_2 (saturation of oxygen in mixed venous blood) value was determined in the Blood Laboratory from this blood sample. For the first two hours after her transfer to ICU, the patient's therapy included a standard postoperative umbrella therapy, discussed in Chapter 4.1, including moderate volume expansion, positive inotropic support and afterload reduction.

The patient was attached to HOTMAN™ System at 12:55. The first data were obtained at 12:56 (Figs.8.1 and 8.2).

As a result of open-chest and open-heart surgery, the patient is at this time dysrhythmic, hemodiluted (Hgb = 9.6 g/dl) and has an elevated level of thoracic fluids (TFC), as expected. Since the invasively measured pressures (CVP and PAOP) and SvO_2 values were available, the HOTMAN™ System was switched to operate in the **AH mode,** enabling the clinician to enter via the System's keyboard the measured values of these parameters, i.e., CVP = 18 Torr, PAOP = 17 Torr, Hgb = 9.6 g/dl and SvO_2 = 74%. As a result, the System could process and display the **exact** values of SSVRI and LSWI (see Eqs.4.4 and 4.5) and **complete oxygen transport dynamics data** (including the oxygen consumption).

The CI values measured by the thermodilution catheter and CI values measured by the HOTMAN™ System were in good clinical agreement.

Fig.8.1 shows the System's **Monitoring Page at 12:56.** Since the patient underwent a **major surgery** and is approximately **three hours after the surgery**, she qualified for the **POSTOPERATIVE Therapeutic Goal** (see the discussion in Chapter 2), requiring a supranormal level of oxygen delivery. The HOTMAN™ System was, therefore, software-switched into the POSTOPERATIVE Therapeutic Goal.

You can see that in spite of standard postoperative therapy, the patient's global blood flow (SI), perfusion blood flow (CI), oxygen transport data (VO_2I and DO_2I) and the parameters of left heart are profoundly compromised.

Please note the dysrhythmia on ECG signal and an elevated level of TEB-measured TFC (Thoracic Fluids Conductivity). Paradoxically, only two parameters (SpO₂ and MAP), monitored in parallel by the patient's monitor, are normal.

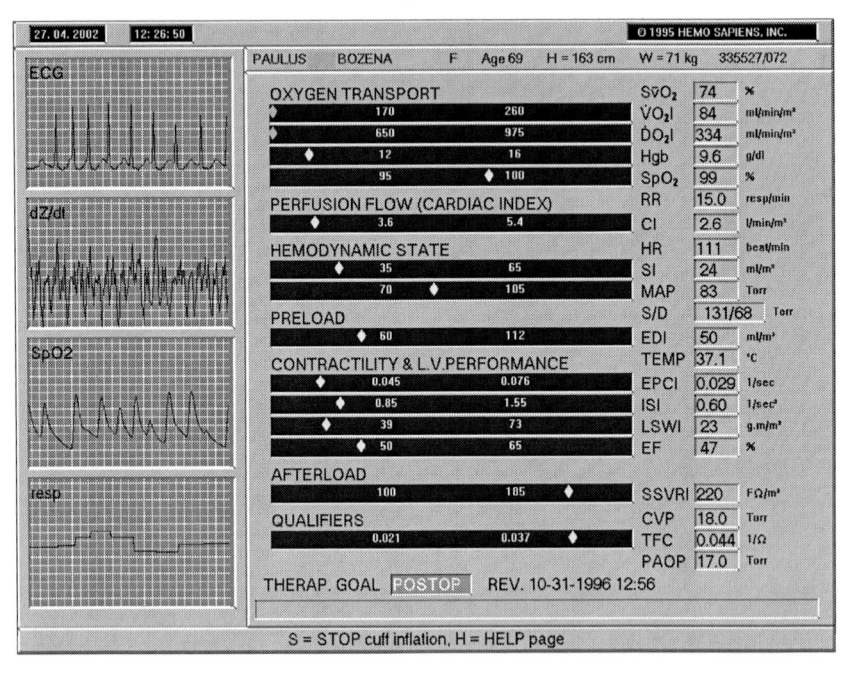

Fig.8.1: Patient's hemodynamic and oxygen transport dynamics status at 12:56 as displayed on the HOTMAN™ F111 System's Monitoring Page. Analog signals of **ECG**, **dZ/dt**, **SpO₂** and **resp** ($\Delta R/\Delta t$ = Rate of respiration over time) are in the left windows. Digital values (including their physical dimensions) of 22 processed TEB, hemodynamic and oxygen transport parameters are on the right. The yellow diamond represents an analog counterpart of the value of each parameter that exhibits a normal range. Normal ranges of these parameters are in form of white numbers within blue strips: The left column of white numbers contains normal minima, the right column normal maxima, specific for gender and age. This graphical feature allows for a very rapid identification of parameters, which are normal, which are supranormal and which are infranormal. Note the System is switched into the Postoperative Therapeutic Goal.

Fig.8.2 represents the **Hemodynamic Management Page** of the System, which is the computer's interpretation of the Hemodynamic Management Chart (Fig.5.5). The data are from the same time slot as in Fig.8.1 - at 12:56.

Compare SI & MAP values in Fig.8.1 with the position of the patient's hemodynamic point in Fig.8.2.

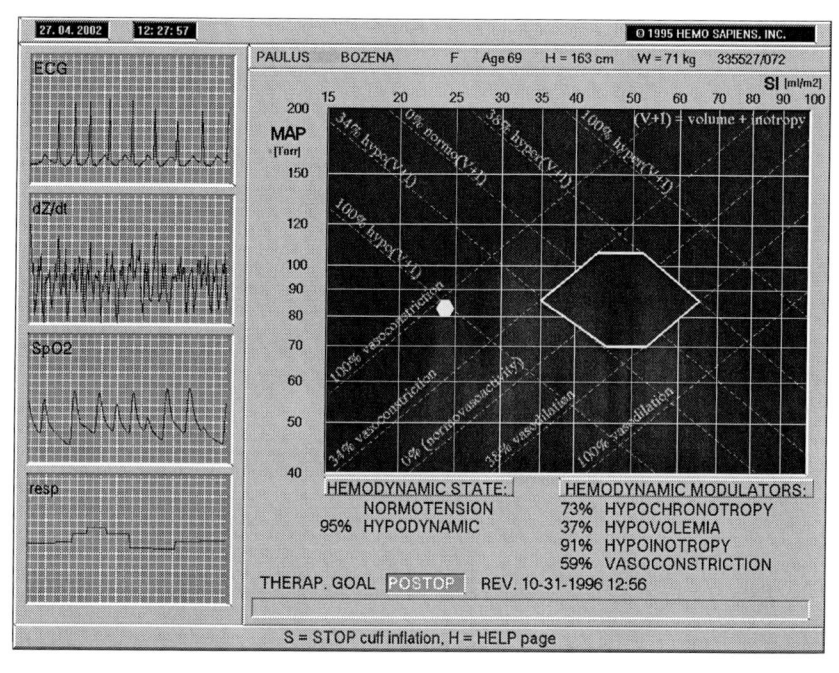

Fig.8.2: Hemodynamic Management Page of the System, which is the computer's interpretation of the Hemodynamic Management Chart (Fig.5.5). Patient's hemodynamic state is expressed graphically by the position of yellow hexagon within the hemodynamic state map (SI & MAP), and verbally under the heading HEMODYNAMIC STATE. Status of patient's hemodynamic modulators is expressed graphically by the position of yellow hexagon within the coordinates of hemodynamic modulators (diagonal isolines of SSVRI and LCWI) and verbally under heading HEMODYNAMIC MODULATORS, including the status of chronotropy (see Chapter 5.5.1). This data presentation is based upon the same data and in the same time slot as in Fig.8.1.

As you can see from the hemodynamic analysis by the System, though the patient is normotensive and has a normal level of SpO_2, her global blood flow is profoundly compromised (95% hypodynamic). The causes of this hemodynamic state are 37% hypovolemia, 91% hypoinotropy and 59% vasoconstriction. In addition, her perfusion blood flow is compromised as well (73% hypochronotropy).

As a result of this information, the therapy was immediately altered: Rate of volume expansion was slightly increased, level of inotropic support (dopamine) was doubled and level of vasodilators was also doubled.

The real-time capabilities of the system thus allow a more aggressive hemodynamic management approach, since the new position of the hemodynamic point and calculated deviations in hemodynamic modulators are displayed several times a minute. This feature enables the clinician to rapidly correct the deviations and, when their normal levels are reached, change their infusion rates as to **maintain** the desired hemodynamic state.

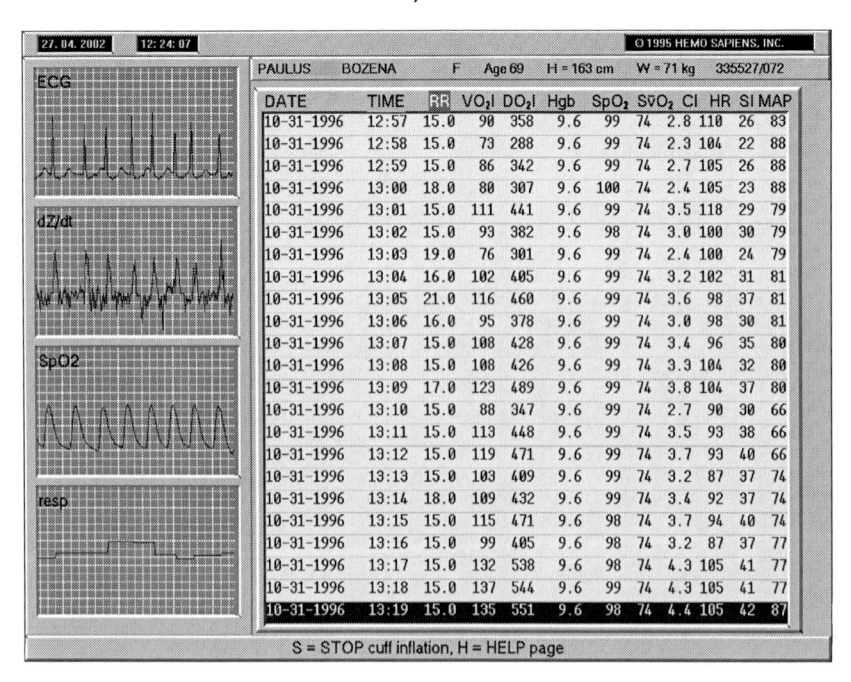

Fig.8.3a: Left half of the **Digital Data Page.** The first two columns are the date and time of recording, followed by the oxygen transport and hemodynamic data. Please note the 1-minute increments in automatic data recordings. Follow significant increases in SI, CI, DO$_2$I and VO$_2$I over the 24-minute period of the normohemodynamic goal-oriented therapy, which included an increased rate of volume expansion, increased rate of positive inotropic support and vasodilatation. Note that RR (Respiratory Rate), HR, SpO$_2$ and MAP – parameters monitored by current patient monitors – are not showing any profound changes during the same time. Fig.8.3b displays the right half of the Digital Data Page.

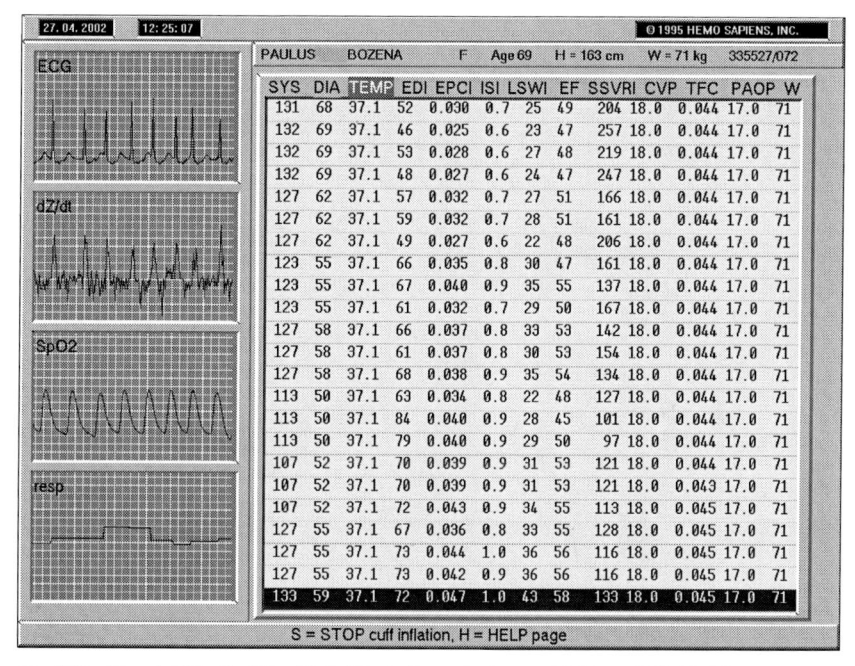

SYS	DIA	TEMP	EDI	EPCI	ISI	LSWI	EF	SSVRI	CVP	TFC	PAOP	W
131	68	37.1	52	0.030	0.7	25	49	204	18.0	0.044	17.0	71
132	69	37.1	46	0.025	0.6	23	47	257	18.0	0.044	17.0	71
132	69	37.1	53	0.028	0.6	27	48	219	18.0	0.044	17.0	71
132	69	37.1	48	0.027	0.6	24	47	247	18.0	0.044	17.0	71
127	62	37.1	57	0.032	0.7	27	51	166	18.0	0.044	17.0	71
127	62	37.1	59	0.032	0.7	28	51	161	18.0	0.044	17.0	71
127	62	37.1	49	0.027	0.6	22	48	206	18.0	0.044	17.0	71
123	55	37.1	66	0.035	0.8	30	47	161	18.0	0.044	17.0	71
123	55	37.1	67	0.040	0.9	35	55	137	18.0	0.044	17.0	71
123	55	37.1	61	0.032	0.7	29	50	167	18.0	0.044	17.0	71
127	58	37.1	66	0.037	0.8	33	53	142	18.0	0.044	17.0	71
127	58	37.1	61	0.037	0.8	30	53	154	18.0	0.044	17.0	71
127	58	37.1	68	0.038	0.9	35	54	134	18.0	0.044	17.0	71
113	50	37.1	63	0.034	0.8	22	48	127	18.0	0.044	17.0	71
113	50	37.1	84	0.040	0.9	28	45	101	18.0	0.044	17.0	71
113	50	37.1	79	0.040	0.9	29	50	97	18.0	0.044	17.0	71
107	52	37.1	70	0.039	0.9	31	53	121	18.0	0.044	17.0	71
107	52	37.1	70	0.039	0.9	31	53	121	18.0	0.043	17.0	71
107	52	37.1	72	0.043	0.9	34	55	113	18.0	0.045	17.0	71
127	55	37.1	67	0.036	0.8	33	55	128	18.0	0.045	17.0	71
127	55	37.1	73	0.044	1.0	36	56	116	18.0	0.045	17.0	71
127	55	37.1	73	0.042	0.9	36	56	116	18.0	0.045	17.0	71
133	59	37.1	72	0.047	1.0	43	58	133	18.0	0.045	17.0	71

S = STOP cuff inflation, H = HELP page

Fig.8.3b: The right half of the Digital Data Page between 12:56 and 13:19. Please, note the increase of EDI and EPCI as a result of volume expansion, EPCI and ISI as a result of positive inotropic support, and a decrease in SSVRI as a result of vasodilatation. Since the extravascular thoracic fluids could not change during the 24-minute period, a small but recognizable increase of TFC is attributable to a volume increase in the intravascular space – a result of volume expansion.

Since the System stores on its hard drive the patient's data every minute, Figs.8.3a and 8.3b are the stored patient's data (upper and lower half of data in Fig.8.1) over the 24-minute hemodynamic management period between 12:56 and 13:19.

The results of the normohemodynamic goal-oriented therapy in just 24 minutes are in Fig.8.4 (Hemodynamic Management Page) and Fig.8.5 (Monitoring Page).

The Hemodynamic Management Page at 13:19 (Fig.8.4) clearly shows that when the identified deviations in hemodynamic modulators were therapeutically corrected, the patient became normovolemic, normoinotropic and normovasoactive. These hemodynamic therapeutic corrections were sufficient to increase the global blood flow/beat (SI) by about 68% (the patient became normodynamic), so no chronotropic therapy was needed.

The Monitoring Page at the same time (Fig.8.5) documents complete improvements of the patient's hemodynamics. The only abnormal parameters are TFC (this parameter attains normal level within days after the surgery, when the thoracic fluids are drained and/or absorbed) and DO_2I (attributable to hemodilution [Hgb = 9.6 g/dl]; this deficiency can be corrected by transfusion of packed red blood cells).

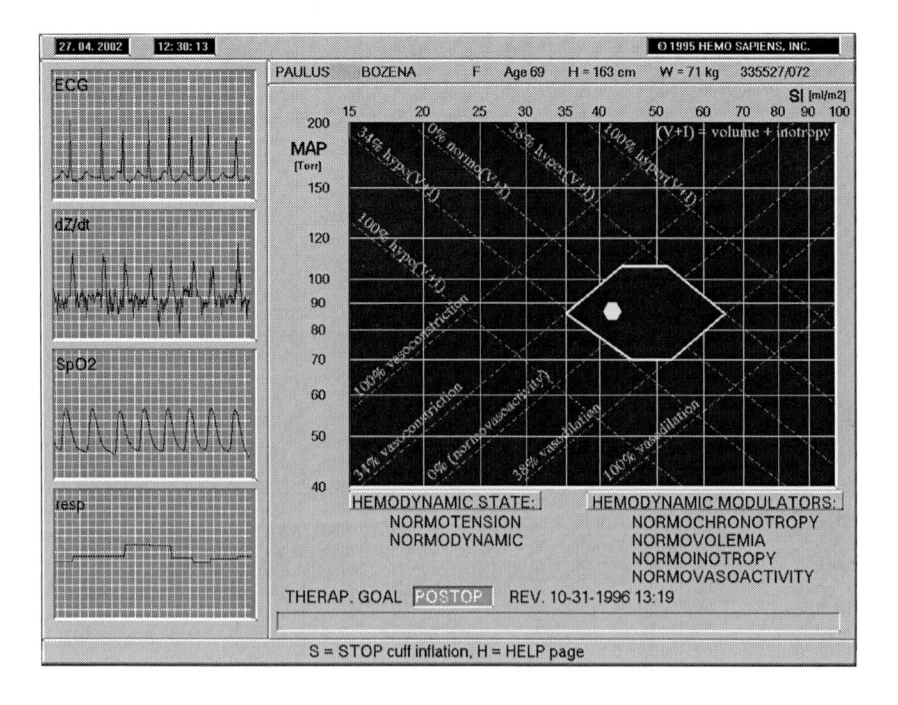

Fig.8.4: Patient's Hemodynamic Management Page at 13:19 after 24 minutes of correct normohemodynamic goal-oriented therapy. See text for explanation.

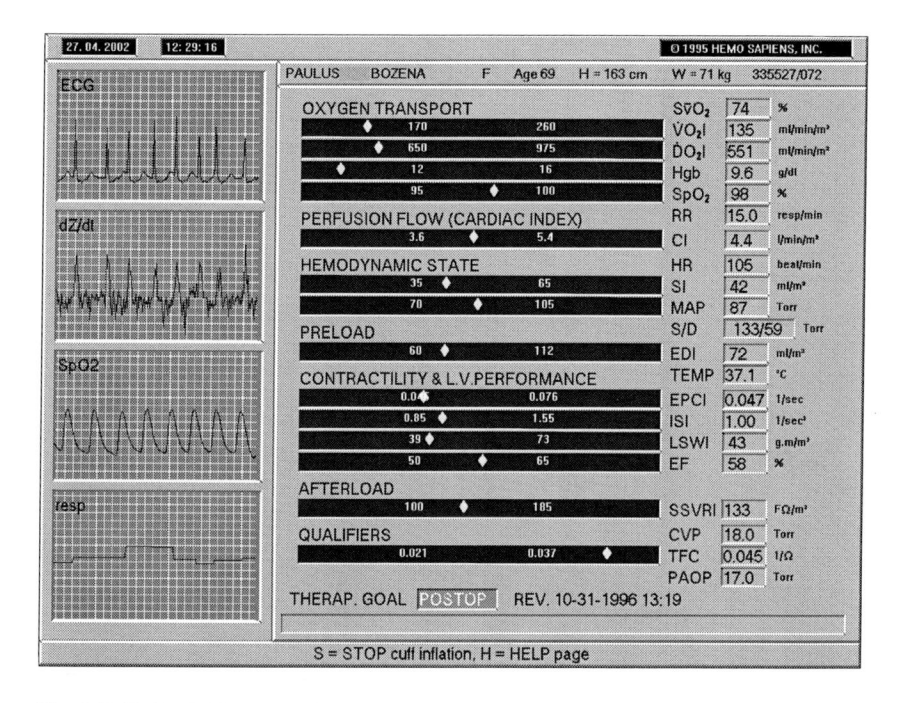

Fig. 8.5: Patient's Monitoring Page at 13:19 after 24 minutes of correct normohemodynamic goal-oriented therapy. See text for explanation.

An interesting feature of the HOTMAN™ System - its **hemodynamic management modeling** capability - is documented in Fig.8.6 below. The hemodynamic modeling was performed on the initial hemodynamic state at 12:56, documented by position of the yellow hemodynamic point (compare to Fig.8.1). During the hemodynamic modeling, the clinician can "administer" any cardio- and/or vasoactive agent in "low," "medium" or "high" dose, without exposing the patient to potentially harmful consequences of an incorrectly selected therapy. "A low dose" corresponds to deviations <40% (do not forget, the normal range of each modulator is up to ± 20% of deviation), "medium dose" to deviations 40-60%, and "high dose" if the deviation in corresponding hemodynamic or perfusion flow modulator exceeds 60%.

The hemodynamic modeling on this patient shows a good agreement between the results of actual therapy (Fig.8.4) and modeling, indicating that this patient's causes of abnormal hemodynamics were clearly of hemodynamic nature only.

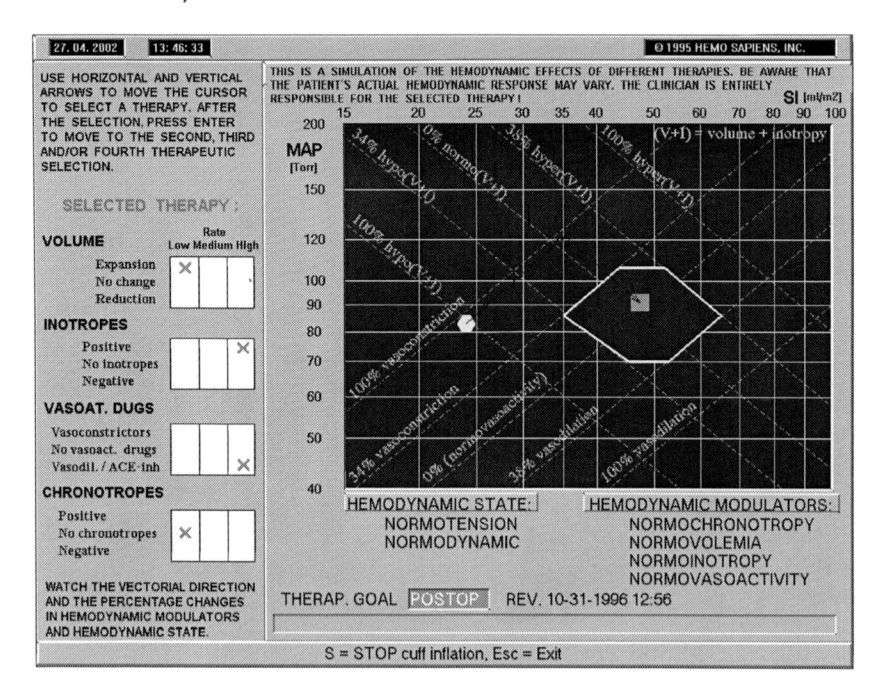

Fig.8.6: Hemodynamic Modeling feature of the HOTMAN™ System: The clinician can "administer" any cardio- and/or vasoactive agent in "low," "medium" or "high" dose, without exposing the patient to potentially harmful consequences of an incorrectly selected therapy. "A low dose" corresponds to a displayed deviation <40%, "medium dose" to deviation 40-60%, and "high dose" if the deviation in corresponding hemodynamic or perfusion flow modulator exceeds 60%. This modeling shows a good clinical agreement with the results of actual hemodynamic management in Fig.8.4.

8.2. Hemodynamic Management of a Hypertensive Patient

The per-beat hemodynamic management method is applicable not only in the critical care setting, as documented in the preceding case study, but its use in treatment of hypertension can have a profound impact on national health care: Cardiovascular diseases are still the leading causes of mortalities in most of the industrialized countries. Hypertension is the contributing factor - about every third middle age adult is hypertensive. Unfortunately, not every hypertensive is treated and, in the treated subgroup, the outcomes of antihypertensive therapy are poor:

NIH (National Institute of Health)[19] and drug manufacturers provide guidelines for selection of antihypertensive drug(s). Current hemodynamic goal is to reduce the blood pressure to a normotensive level. Last NIH Report[19], covering the period 1991-94, lists the following outcome-related US numbers: 53.6% of hypertensives were treated, out of which 27.4% had their hypertension controlled (i.e., 72.6% of treated hypertensives remained hypertensive in spite of taking antihypertensive medications).

It should now be clear to a reader of this textbook that poor outcomes in treatment of hypertension are mostly related to current methodology, which, rather than identifying and treating the patient-specific causes (hypervolemia, hyperinotropy and vasoconstriction), treats the symptom (hypertension), while disregarding the need for adequate perfusion in treated hypertensives. Digestive disorders, male impotence, tiredness, sleepwalking, body temperature control problems, etc., are often labeled as "side-effects of antihypertensive therapy," while they are, in many cases, clear clinical expressions of a low flow state.

First significant study on use of per-beat hemodynamic for treatment of hypertension, reporting significant improvements in outcomes, was presented at the 11th Scientific Meeting of The American Society of Hypertension, New York, NY, 1996.

A condensed transcript of this paper follows:

NORMOHEMODYNAMIC GOAL-ORIENTED ANTIHYPERTENSIVE THERAPY IMPROVES THE OUTCOME

Sramek BB, Int'l Hemodynamic Society, USA
Tichy JA, Hojerova M, Cervenka V
Institute for Preventive Care, Prague, Czech Republic

Normohemodynamic state involves a simultaneous normotension and normodynamic circulation. A noninvasive measurement of cardiac output and the hemodynamic management chart, which identifies the causes of abnormal hemodynamics (the percentage deviations in volume, inotropy, vasoactivity and chronotropy from their normal levels), were added to the noninvasive armament for treatment of hypertension and implemented into a hemodynamic assessment, monitoring and management system (HOTMAN® F111 System, HEMO SAPIENS INC.). Instead of a conventional selection of antihypertensive drugs by trial-and-error, we were able to identify and administer such antihypertensive drug(s), which were optimal and specific for each patient.

383 randomly selected hypertensive patients (230 men and 153 women), previously treated by a conventional therapy of at least 2 antihypertensive drugs between 2 and 42 years (mean 12.5 years), were used in the study.

A scattergram of hemodynamic points of all patients at the onset of the study is in Fig. 8.7.

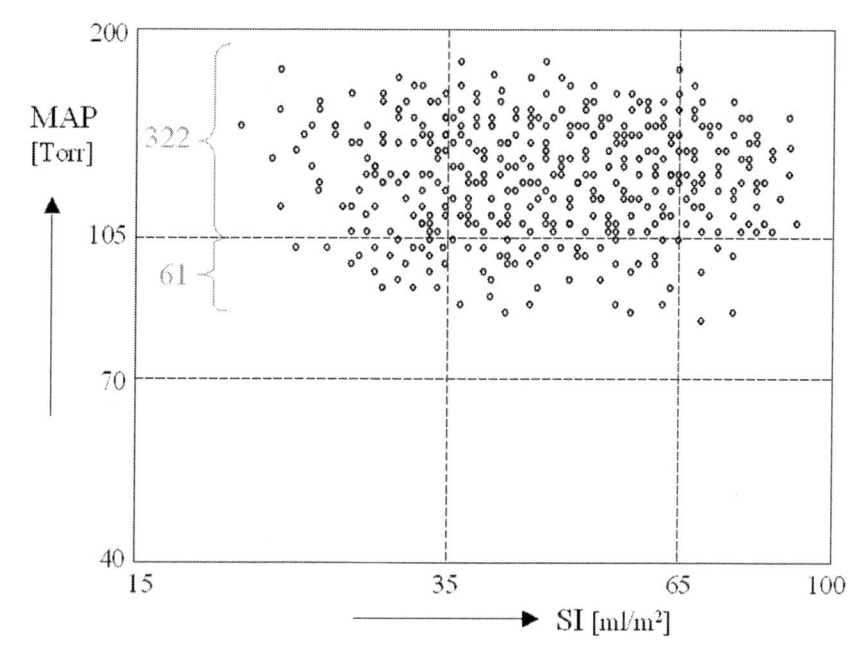

Fig. 8.7: Scattergram of hemodynamic points of all 383 patients measured at the onset of the study

During the initial noninvasive hemodynamic assessment, 61 patients (15.9%) had their blood pressure within the normotensive range (MAP < 105 Torr) and were excluded from a further participation in the study.

The remaining 322 patients covered mild, moderate and severe hypertension categories. 51 of these (15.8%) were hypodynamic hypertensives, 210 (65.2%) were normodynamic hypertensives and 61 (18.9%) were hyperdynamic hypertensives. Scattergram of hemodynamic points of these 322 patients who remained hypertensive in spite of using at least 2 antihypertensive drugs for at least 2 years is in Fig.8.8.

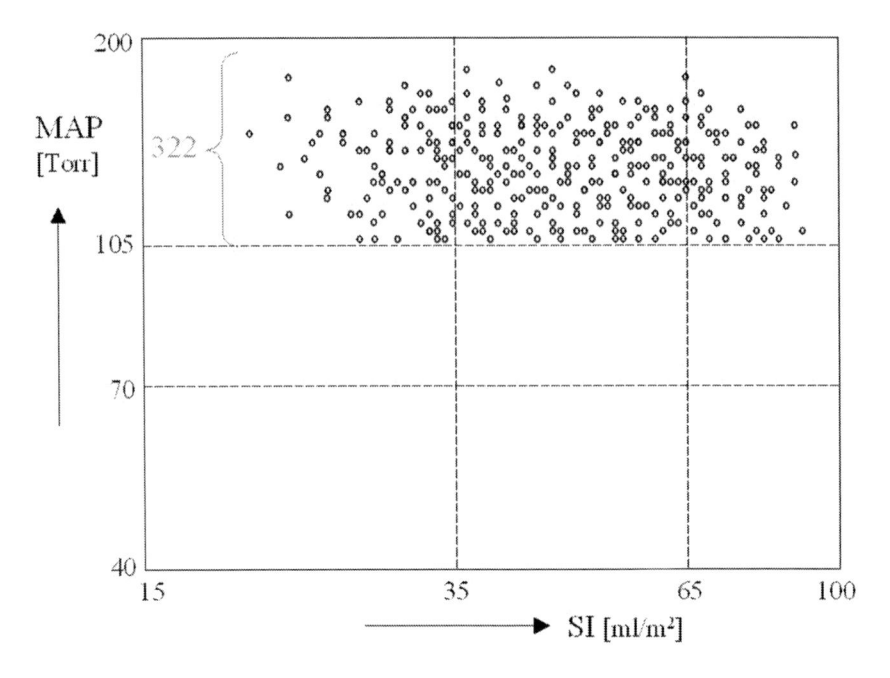

Fig.8.8: Scattergram of hemodynamic points of 322 patients who remained hypertensive with conventional antihypertensive therapy in spite of using at least 2 antihypertensive drugs for at least 2 years

All these 322 hypertensives were then prescribed antihypertensive drugs, which generic categories were suggested by the System, as to aim for both normotension and normodynamic state.

All patients were measured again in approximately 3 weeks. Though normotension could not be achieved by a conventional antihypertensive therapy in any of these 322 patients, the normohemodynamic goal-oriented therapy produced normotension in 203 of them (63%). In addition, 242 patients (75%) became normodynamic. Scattergram of hemodynamic points of these 322 patients after three weeks of normohemodynamic goal-oriented therapy is in Fig.8.9. This profound hemodynamic improvement took place in the first therapeutic intervention.

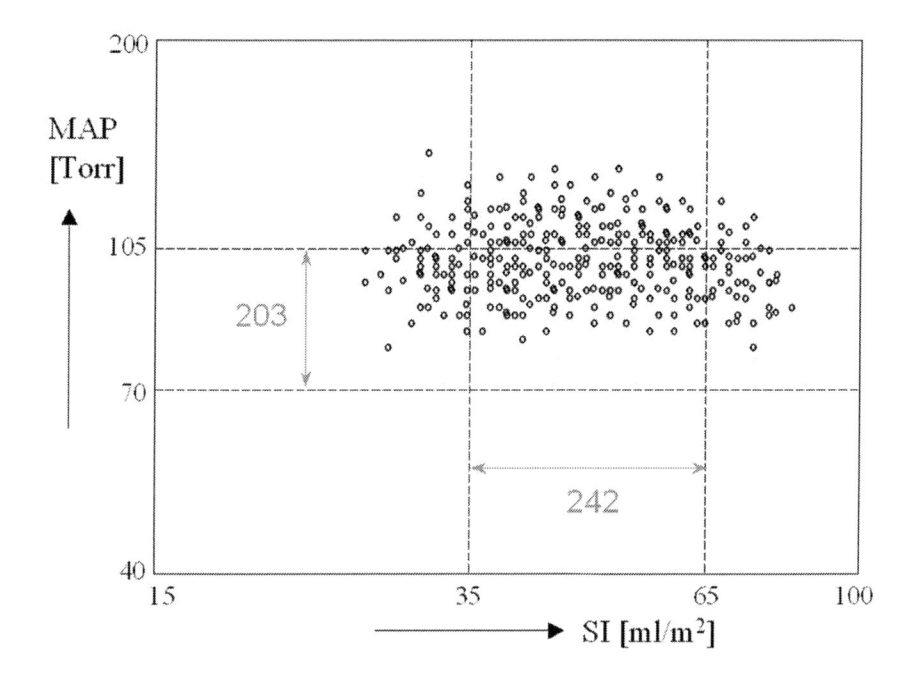

Fig.8.9: Scattergram of hemodynamic points of these 322 patients after three weeks of normohemodynamic goal-oriented therapy

8.1.1. Management of a Hypertensive Patient: A Case Study

Etiology of hypertension is fairly complex, however, there is enough evidence that a significant majority of hypertension is of hemodynamic origin and, as a result, can be successfully treated by identifying its causes and administering therapy, which negates the effects of the hemodynamic causes. The therapeutic goal for treatment of hypertension **must be both normotension and normohemodynamic and normoperfusion states.** The following case study is documenting exactly that. The data have been provided courtesy of HEMO SAPIENS® INC.

A 70-year old male had been hypertensive for about 20 years at the time of his first measurement by the HOTMAN™ System on June 16, 1999. His hypertension was initially treated with diuretics and, subsequently with beta-blockers. With these therapeutic choices, his quality of life was negatively affected. As a result, his antihypertensive therapy compliance was poor.

The patient's hemodynamics and oxygen transport dynamics were measured first by the HOTMAN™ F111 System on June 16, 1999. The Monitoring Page is in Fig.8.10.

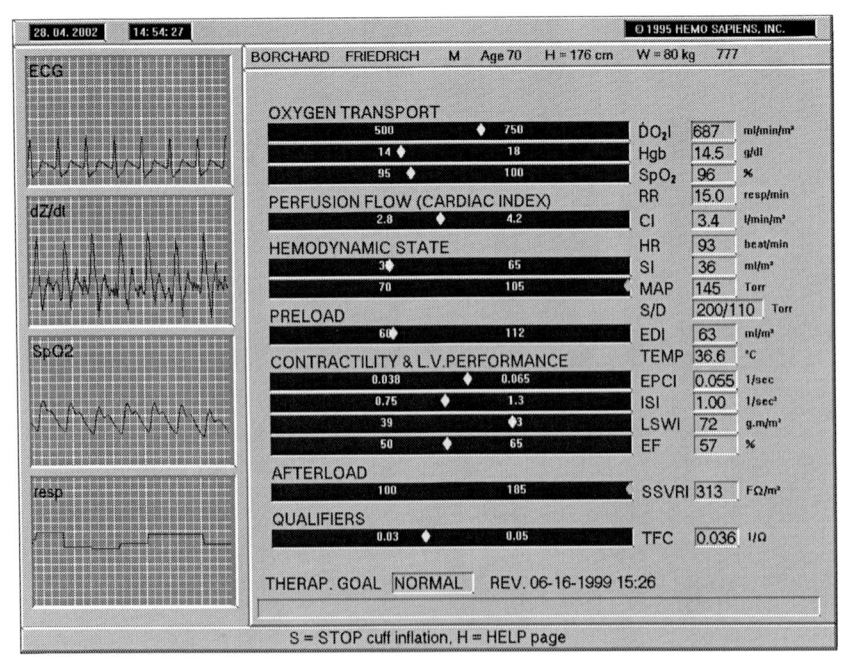

Fig.8.10: Hemodynamic and O_2 transport data of a 70 year old hypertensive male. The patient is borderline normodynamic, profoundly hypertensive, however, due to chronotropic compensation of HR, his perfusion blood flow and O_2 transport are normal.

At this time, the patient is profoundly hypertensive, borderline normodynamic, however, due to a correct chronotropic compensation by HR, his perfusion blood flow and O_2 transport are normal. As a result, even if untreated, his quality of life would be unaffected, though his risk factors would be increased.

The Hemodynamic Management Page at the same time (Fig.8.11) clearly identifies the causes of his hypertension:

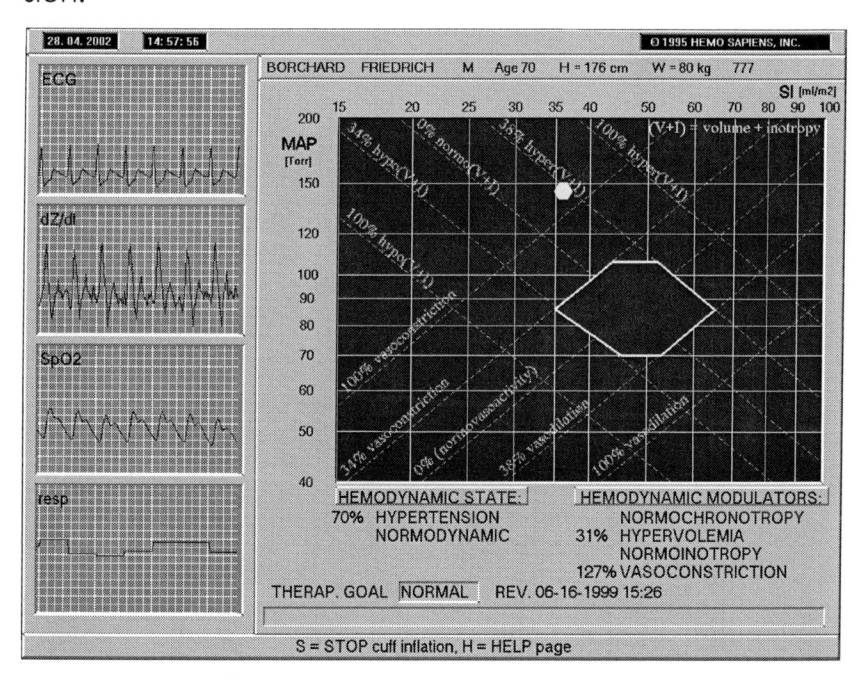

Fig.8.11: The Hemodynamic Management Page corresponding to Fig.8.10. The patient's 70% hypertension is caused by 31% hypervolemia in conjunction with 127% vasoconstriction. Please note the hemodynamic effects of beta-blockers on this patient, modeled in Fig.8.12.

The patient's 70% hypertension is caused by a 31% hypervolemia in conjunction with a 127% vasoconstriction. The diuretics, prescribed to him first, treated only the secondary cause (hypervolemia), while, neither diuretics nor beta-blockers addressed the primary cause of his hypertension – the 127% vasoconstriction. Hemodynamic modeling of beta-blockers in Fig.8.12 is showing why his quality of life was so negatively affected by beta-blocker therapy when it was selected as a replacement for diuretics:

Beta-blockers (negative inotropes + negative chronotropes) treated neither his hypervolemia nor his vasoconstriction, however, changed his normoinotropy to hypoinotropy and normochronotropy to hypochronotropy. After the beta-blocker therapy, instead of having **two** hemodynamic and perfusion state modulators at abnormal level, the patient then had **all four** hemodynamic modulators at abnormal levels:

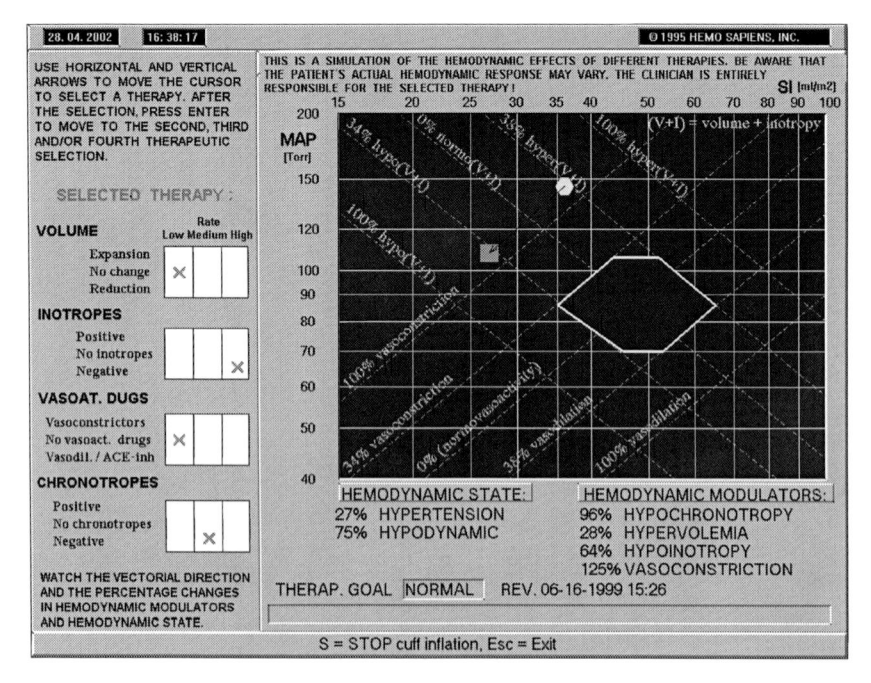

Fig.8.12 - Hemodynamic Modeling: Predicted hemodynamic response of hypertensive patient in Fig.8.11 to beta-blockers. Though lowering his blood pressure, they also lowered his blood flow. Their negative inotropic + negative chronotropic effect treated neither the documented hypervolemia nor vasoconstriction, however, converted two remaining hemodynamic causes, which were initially normal, to profoundly compromised ones.

Based upon identification of hemodynamic modulators responsible for his abnormal hemodynamic state in Fig.8.11 (31% hypervolemia + 127% vasoconstriction), the patient was prescribed a small dose of diuretics and a large dose of ACE-Inhibitors.

In Fig.8.13 is the patient's Hemodynamic Management Page recorded during a medical check-up 2 months later. You can see that selection of a therapy, which treated the causes of his abnormal hemodynamics produced the desired normohemodynamic and normoperfusion states.

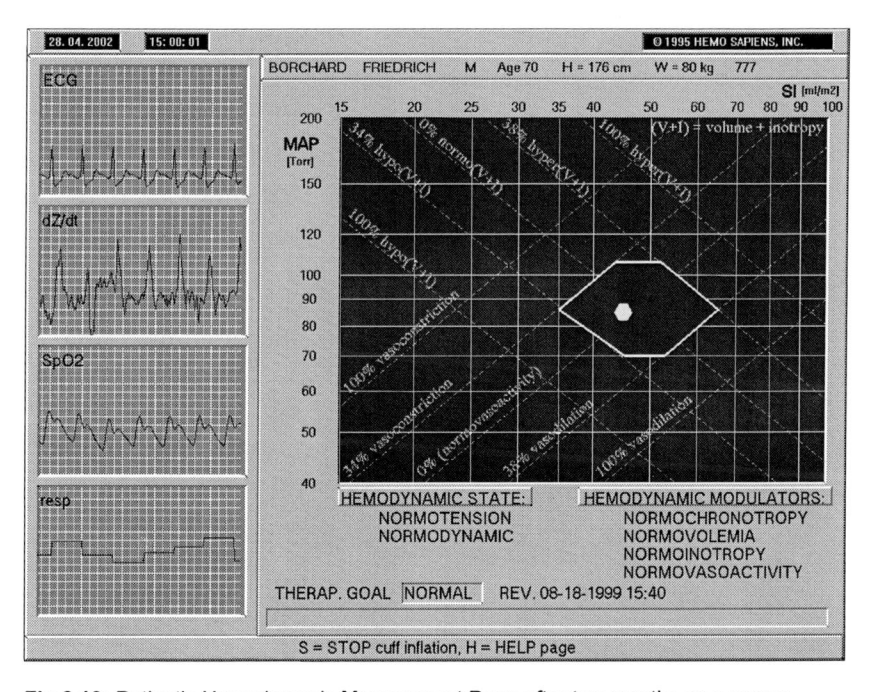

Fig.8.13: Patient's Hemodynamic Management Page after two months on a normohemodynamic goal oriented therapy consisting of a small dose of diuretics and large dose of ACE inhibitors.

Corresponding Monitoring Page after 2 months of normohemodynamic goal oriented therapy is in Fig.8.14. Note that oxygen delivery dynamics, perfusion blood flow and hemodynamic parameters are within their respective normal ranges.

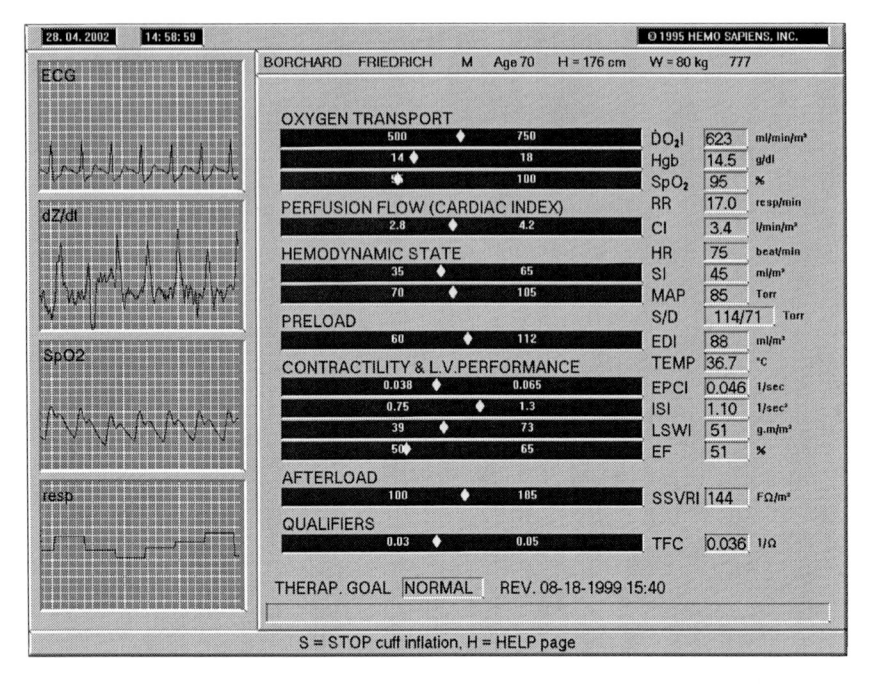

Fig.8.14: Patient's Monitoring Page after two months on a normohemodynamic goal oriented therapy consisting of a small dose of diuretics and large dose of ACE inhibitors.

As it could be expected, the reported patient's quality of life was good.

References

(1) Braunwald E: Assessment of cardiac function. Heart Disease, A Textbook of cardiovascular Medicine. Braunwald E (Ed), Philadelphia, WB Saunders Co., 1984: 467

(2) Milnor WR: Hemodynamics. Williams & Wilkins, 1982: 136&155

(3) Hurst JW: The Heart, McGraw Hill, 1966: 93

(4) Sramek BB: Hemodynamics and its role in oxygen transport. Biomechanics of the Cardiovascular System, 1995, Czech Technical University Press: 209-231

(5) Shoemaker WC, Bland RD, Appel PL: Therapy of Critically Ill Postoperative Patients Based on Outcome Prediction and Prospective Clinical Trials; The Surgical Clinics of North America, August 1985, Critical Care: 811

(6) Levett JM, Replogle RL: Thermodilution Cardiac Output: A Critical Analysis and Review of the Literature. J of Surg Res 27: 392-404, 1979

(7) Calvin JE et al: Does the pulmonary capillary wedge pressure predict left ventricular preload in critically ill patients? Crit Care Med, Vol 9, No 6: 437

(8) Pesce RR: The Swan-Ganz Catheter: It Goes through Your Pulmonary Artery and You Pay through the Nose (Editorial) Resp Care, Sep 89 Vol 34 No 9: 785

(9) Robin ED: The Cult of Swan-Ganz Catheter. Intens & Crit Care Digest, Vol.5, No.1, June 1986: 18

(10) Robin ED: Death by Pulmonary Artery Flow-Directed Catheter *(Editorial)* Time for a Moratorium? Chest/92/4/October 1987

(11) Sramek BB. Hemodynamic and Pump-performance Monitoring by Electrical Bioimpedance - New Concepts. Problems in Respiratory Care, 1989, Vol.2, No.2: 274-290

(12) Sramek BB. Thoracic electrical bioimpedance: Basic principles and physiologic relationship. Noninvas Cardiol 1994;3(2): 83-88

(13) Bernstein DP: Noninvasive Cardiac Output Measurement. Textbook of Crit Care, 1989, WB Saunders: 159-185

(14) Jacobsen B, Webster JG: Medicine and Clinical Engineering, 1977, Prentice-Hall Inc., 1977: 388

(15) Capan LM, et al: Measurement of ejection fraction by bioimpedance method. Crit Care Med 1987;15: 402

(16) Bland JM, Altman DG: Statistical Methods for Assessing Agreement Between Two Methods of Clinical Measurement. The Lancet, Feb.8, 1986: 307

(17) Van Grondelle A, et al: Thermodilution method overestimates low cardiac output in humans. Am J Physiol 1983;245: H690

(18) Sramek BB: Hemodynamics and Pump-performance Monitoring by Electrical Bioimpedance: New Concepts. Problems in Respiratory Care. Vol.2, No.2. April-June 1989: 274-290. J.B. Lippincott Co.

(19) The Sixth Report of the Joint National Committee on Prevention, Detection, Evaluation, and Treatment of High Blood Pressure. NIH, No.98-43080, November 1997

(20) Weissler AM et al: Systolic time intervals in heart failure in man. Circulation, Vol.37, No.2, 1968: 149

(21) Stein PD, Sabbah HN: Force-velocity-length relations in man expressed by a single hemodynamic expression: The ejection rate of change of power at peak tension. Amer J of Cardiol, Vol.37, 1976: 871

(22) Penaz J: Mayer Waves: History and Methodology. Automedica, 1978, Vol.2: 135-141

(23) Sramek BB, Hraska V: Normal Values of Hemodynamic, O_2 Delivery and TEB Parameters in Neonatal and Pediatric Patients. Proceedings of 4th Int'l Conference on Hemodynamics of the International Hemodynamic Society, 1998, Acapulco

(24) Sramek BB, Nouzova K, Parizek A: Normal Values of Hemodynamic, O_2 Delivery and TEB Parameters in Gravidas and Nongravidas. Proceedings of 4th Int'l Conference on Hemodynamics of the International Hemodynamic Society, 1998, Acapulco

Index

Afterload: 38, 61
Bland-Altman's Method: 27
Body Surface Area (BSA): 14, 15
Cardiac Index (CI): 15
    Augmentation: 16
    Normal value: 16
    Postoperative: 19
Cardiac Output (CO): 13
    Normal values in Mammals: 14
Chronotropy: 39
Contractility: 38, 81
    Isovolumic Phase: 54
Correlation coefficient: 27
Central Venous Pressure (CVP): 69
dP/dt: 56
Ejection Fraction: 25, 36
Ejection Phase Contractility Index (EPCI): 24
End-Diastolic Index (EDI): 36
End-Systolic Volume: 60
Filling Pressure: 35
Flow-directed Pulmonary Artery (PA) Catheter: 3
Hemodynamic Data:
    Neonatal & Pediatric Patients: 85
    Gravidas & Nongravidas
Hemodynamic measurement: 3
Hemodynamic Management: 41, 65
    Chart: 75
    Hypertension: 109
    in ICU: 100
    with Per-minute hemodynamics: 41
    with Per-beat hemodynamics: 65Hemodynamic
Map: 65
Hemodynamic Modulation: 33

        Chronotropy: 62
        Inotropy: 71
        Intravascular Volume: 53, 71
        Mechanical & Pharmacological: 54
        Vasoactivity: 61, 67
        Timing considerations: 64
Hemodynamic Responses: 78
Hemodynamics: 3, 33
Hemodynamics – definition: 10
Hyperinotropy: 59, 80
Hyperchronotropy: 62, 83
Hypervolemia: 54, 82
Hypochronotropy: 62, 84
Hypoinotropy: 59, 80
Hypovolemia: 54, 82
Inotropic State Index (ISI): 25, 58
        Measure: 56, 57
Inotropy: 58, 80
Left Cardiac Work Index (LCWI): 40
Left Stroke Work Index (LSWI): 52
Mayer Waves: 48
Mean Arterial Pressure (MAP): 11
Normochronotropy: 62, 84
Normohemodynamic State: 66
Normoinotropy: 56, 80
Normovasoactivity: 61, 83
Normovolemia: 53, 82
Outcomes: 3
Oxygen Transport: 30
Oxygen Delivery (DO_2): 13, 30
        Index (DO_2I): 15
Oxygen Consumption Index (VO_2I): 30
Patient monitors: 4
Peak Aortic Blood Flow Acceleration (PABA): 57
Preload: 35
Perfusion Blood Flow: 62

Pulmonary Artery Occluded Pressure (PAOP): 10, 21, 34, 43
    and blood volume: 10, 21
Sramek's Equation: 25
Stewart-Hamilton Equation: 21
Stroke Volume (SV): 11
Stroke Index (SI): 16
    Augmentation: 16
    Normal value: 16
Stroke Systemic Vascular Resistance Index (SSVRI): 49
Survival: 17
Systemic hemodynamics: 10
Systemic Vascular Resistance (SVR): 39
    Index (SVRI): 39
Systolic Time Intervals: 56
Thermodilution (TD) technique/method: 20
Thoracic Electrical Bioimpedance (TEB): 22
    Signal: 23
    Clinical agreement with TD: 28
Vasoactivity: 82
Vasoconstriction: 61, 83
Vasodilation: 61, 83